BOBBI BROWN BEAUTY

THE ULTIMATE BEAUTY RESOURCE

BOBBI BROWN BEAUTY

THE ULTIMATE BEAUTY RESOURCE BOBBI BROWN & ANNEMARIE IVERSON

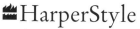HarperStyle

An Imprint of CollinsPublishers
A Division of HarperCollins*Publishers*

Photography credits appear on page 242.

HarperCollins books may be purchased for educational, business, or sales promotional use. For information please write: Special Markets Department, HarperCollins Publishers, Inc., 10 East 53rd Street, New York, NY 10022.

FIRST EDITION

Designed by Shahid & Company

Library of Congress Cataloging-in-Publication Data
Brown, Bobbi
    Bobbi Brown beauty / Bobbi Brown and Annemarie Iverson.—1st ed.
    ISBN 0-06-270167-3
    1. Beauty, Personal.   I. Iverson, Annemarie.   II. Title.
    RA778.B669 1997   96-23880
    646.7'42—dc20

97 98 99 00 01 ◆/F 10 9 8 7

Printed in Canada

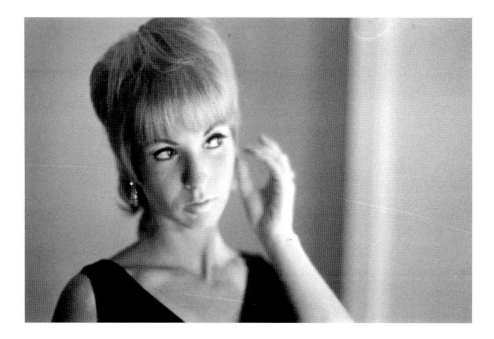

To my mother, Sandra Cain, who, from my earliest days, intrigued and inspired me with her glamour, her beauty rituals, her white shadow, and her pale, pale lips. Also, to the men in my life: my wonderful husband, Steven, my two boys, Dylan and Dakota, and my dad, James Brown. They make me whole.

ACKNOWLEDGMENTS

Bobbi and Annemarie thank Patricia Van der Leun for her calm and encouragement throughout this project, Diane Reverand for her enthusiasm for the book and confidence in us; Ilan Rubin and Troy Word for their beautiful photographs; and Jessica Weinstein for her tireless work in gathering photographs and staging photography shoots for this book. In addition, the authors and Jessica acknowledge with gratitude the generous contributions of the following individuals:

Michel and Linda Arnaud, Nancy Assunsao, Bryan Bantry, Delores Barrett, Gilles Bensimon, Kelly Bloom, Rachel Bold for The Gap, Jill Bredel, Janine Cappiello, Walter Chin, Michel Comte, Elizabeth Costa for American Models, Creighton for Robert Kree, Patrick Demarchelier, Suzanne Donaldson, Suzanne Donovan for Ford, Sante D'Orazio, Meaghan Dowling, Arthur Elgort, Betty Eng, Carlos Frederico Farina, Sara Foley Anderson, Gene Goldberg, Dennis Golonka, Myra Gonzalez and Stuart Ross at IMG Models, Kara Glynn for Industria Superstudio, Dayle Haddon, Scott Hagendorf for LTI, Rob Hallie for RGH, Patti Hansen, Alan Hardy, Jennifer Harris, Patti Harris for Grey Advertising, Joyce Hartenstein, Ron Hill, Mel Hughes for Studio One, Kristin Ingersoll, Jody Jarel, Janet Johnson, Michael Johnson for Marek, Karen Johnston, Christine Karl, Jean Gabriel Kauss, Viviane Kelly for Michael Kors, Harry King for Kramer & Kramer, Kelly Klein, Brigitte Lacombe, Rosalind Landis, Jeff Licata, Robert Magnotta and Kristy Engels for Edge, Maria McCauley, Alex McElwaine for Rogers & Cowan, Regina Maguire, Lorraine Mead for Condé Nast Publications, Sheila Metzner, Alison Morley, Debra Moses for Vera Wang, Michelle Ocampo, Eric Petersen, Curtis Phelps, Jennifer Preuss, Susan Price for Price Inc., Ken Robinson; Paul Rowland, Jennifer Ramey, Jennifer Borak for Women; Francesco Scavullo, Peter Schlosse, Nancy Seltzer & Associates, Sam Shahid, Laura Shanahan, Jordan Shippenberg, Jennifer Schram for TSE Cashmere, Candy Singer, Sixty Eight Degrees, Inc., Jeff Sowardes, Michelle Thomas for Pauline's, Paul Thomas, Liz Tilberis, John Turner, Ernesto Urdaneta, Antoine Verglas, Bruce Weber, Jackie Weihs, Linda Wells, Peter Wert, and Reid Williams.

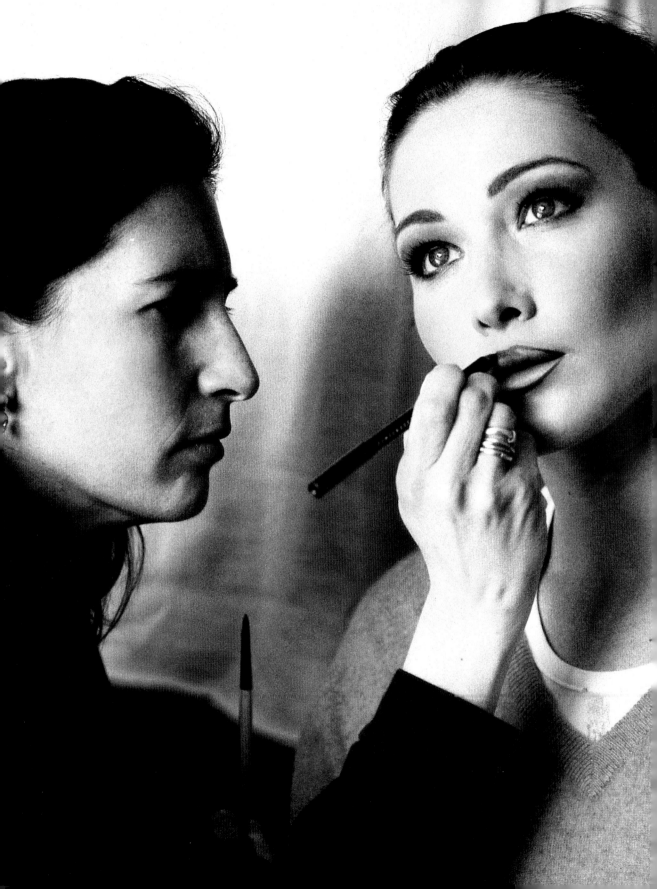

CONTENTS

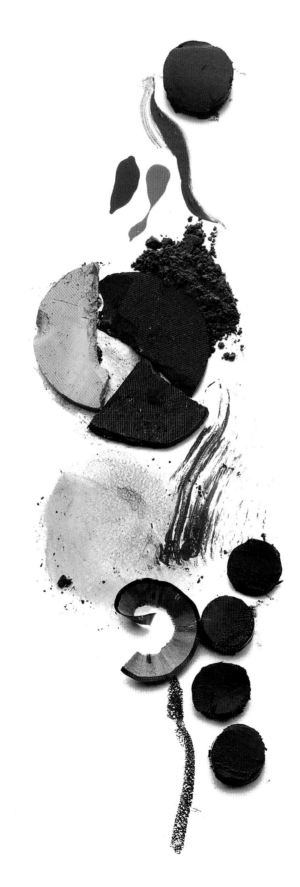

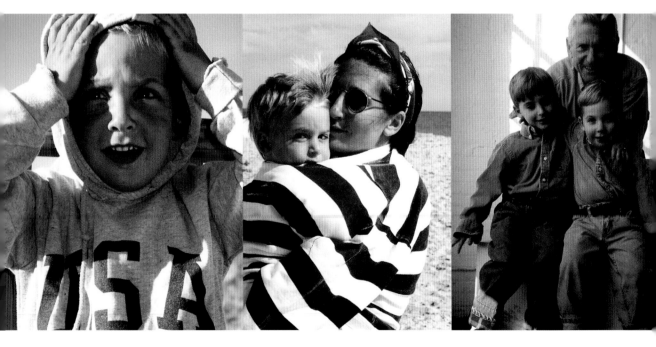

BOBBI'S BIO
BY BOBBI'S FATHER, JAMES BROWN

It is incredible for me to think that my daughter Bobbi Brown has accomplished so much in so little time—it boggles my mind, really, since it feels like so short a time since she was born.

You could say that we grew up together, since I was only twenty-one when Bobbi, my first daughter, was born. We lived in the village of Wilmette, a small suburb north of Chicago. It was in the late 1950s, a peaceful time, I think, to be a child. Looking back, I remember one early incident that, in hindsight, was probably more important than it seemed at the time. When Bobbi was five, she got into her mother's make-up drawer and began applying the makeup to her face, the sink, and the bathroom walls. The lipsticks and rouge were ruined, and Bobbi spent the rest of the afternoon in her bedroom.

Bobbi seemed to pick up two lessons that day: Don't mess with your mama's stuff and playing with makeup is fun. To satisfy our daughter's unabated fascination, we gave Bobbi her very own makeup—lipsticks, brushes, rouges, creams, sponges, powders, and lotions—all slightly used, but perfect for her purposes. Bobbi went at it with the heaviest of hands—it was not a pretty sight.

Experimenting with cosmetics continued to be a passion in her grow-ing years, more as a game than as an exercise in vanity. When it was time to decide on colleges, she sought a university where she could study makeup—theatrical makeup—and pursue her goal of becoming a make-up artist. She first tried a school in Wisconsin for a year, but that institution failed to see the value in her subject. The next one was in Arizona, but she met with the same resistance.

But Bobbi figured things out on her own, finding a school in Boston, Emerson College, that would allow her to major in makeup. I couldn't help but inquire how she would hold up under the stress of a mascara final! But she did it and graduated with a B.F.A. in theatrical makeup.

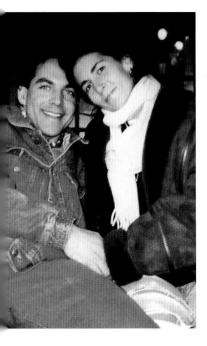

From far left: my son Dakota; on the beach with Dylan; my father with the boys; my husband, Steven Plofker, and I, out west on our honeymoon.

After graduation, Bobbi knew that she would have only one shot at making it, and that Boston wasn't the place to be. She didn't know a single person in New York City, but she went there anyway. She spent a lot of time trying and plodding and pounding the pavement. When things didn't seem to be working, she would worry and maybe cry a little. That's when I would get a call. Usually, all she needed to hear was "poor baby" and "go get 'em."

Bobbi kept walking around with her portfolio tucked under her arm. She would show it to anyone who would look at it and listen to her—to anyone who would take the time to look. As her experience grew, her talent became more apparent. And the quality of her portfolio became better and better.

Of course, from my vantage point in Chicago, I remained a little skeptical—until I went to a *Vogue* party with Bobbi during a visit to New York. I was introduced to an editor at that magazine and I asked her whether my daughter was as talented as I'd been hearing. "You don't succeed in this town," she responded, "unless you are more than just talented." That's when I started really believing.

We used to take family vacations in Ocho Rios, Jamaica. To practice and pass the time, Bobbi would enlist her brothers as models for her theatrical makeup. Jeff would be made to look like an old woman. Paul would be made to look like an old man, while Michael came out looking

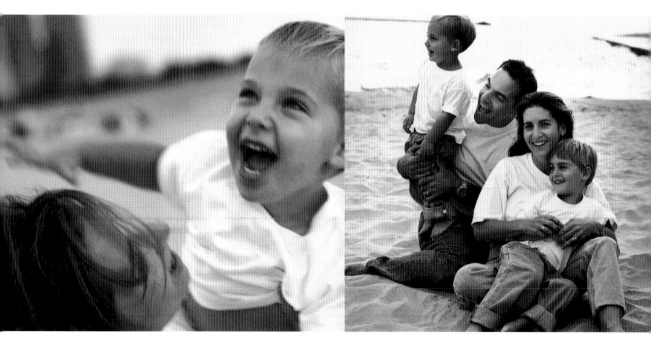

like the loser in the prizefight of the century. Pictures of these experiments still hang in the family photo gallery on the bathroom wall.

So, some twelve years later, it seemed remarkable to me that while the family was again vacationing in Ocho Rios, there was Bobbi a few houses away. This time she was on assignment with Italian *Vogue*, applying makeup to the beautiful faces of Yasmeen Ghauri and Helena Christensen, two of the most famous models in the world.

It was around this time that Bobbi—now an accomplished, sought-after makeup artist with access to the best makeup in the world—started to think about the products themselves. To Bobbi, nothing looked natural enough. No matter how you applied the green or blue that was popular at this particular moment in the 1980s, it still looked like makeup. It didn't satisfy her vision of a naturally beautiful woman. She took the best of what was available and mixed and blended. She kept getting closer to the makeup-less look that she loves, but still couldn't get it quite right.

Bobbi consulted with suppliers, chemists, and product colorists to

From lower left: Bobbi and Dakota; Bobbi, Steven, and the boys; Bobbi with the "guys": husband Steven, father James, and sons Dylan and Dakota; Bobbi, Dakota, and Steven.

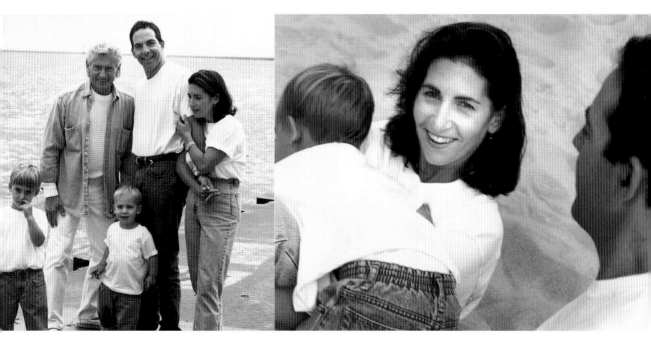

learn what makes what do what. She added this to her practical knowledge and formulated the first lip colors that were the basis of her company, Bobbi Brown Essentials. There were ten lipsticks, numbered one to ten, all slight modulations of nude and natural. That might seem like a humble beginning, but for Bobbi it was exactly what she tried to achieve; they were simple to use and the quality was very, very high.

From what I read in magazines and hear on television, Bobbi's company has since become the quintessential American makeup line for perfectly simple and natural products that don't force women to change their makeup constantly and isn't based on instant obsolescence. She has given American women something that they need, and they have responded by loving it.

All of which is to say that Bobbi is a warm and caring woman before all else—before all of her success and celebrity. She is a loving wife, a nurturing mother, and a considerate friend. While I am proud of her success in business, it pales beside my pride in her as a kind and giving human being.

There is a bottom line to her beliefs: You cannot create beauty. That is God's domain. You can only enhance the beauty that emanates from within. If the body is healthy, the face will glow. Then, with makeup, it's just the touch-up, the fill-in. Bobbi practices what she preaches. She works out constantly, eats healthful foods, and tries to make the rest of us do the same. I am probably the only grandfather in America who has never taken his grandsons out for a hamburger.

Bobbi constantly demonstrates to those she comes into contact with that she will not trade her humanity for fame and fortune. She knows she can have both and keeps both sides of her life in proper perspective. It's a wonderful thing to be her father. Bobbi has given me pride and she has given me Steven, my son-in-law, and Dakota and Dylan, my grandsons.

There is something known as the American Dream—the concept that anyone can rise from humble, obscure beginnings by his or her own powers and attain incredible heights. That is the story of Bobbi Brown (her real and original name, I assure you), whom I dearly love and hope will live happily ever after.

James Brown
March 1996

4

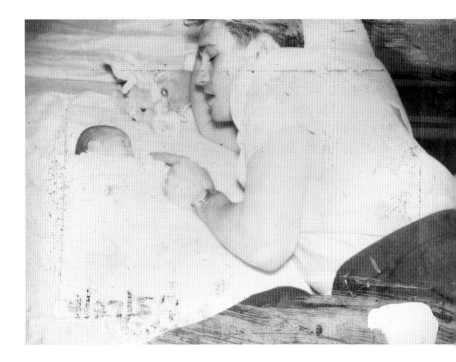

James Brown, age 21, with Bobbi, age 1 week (1957).

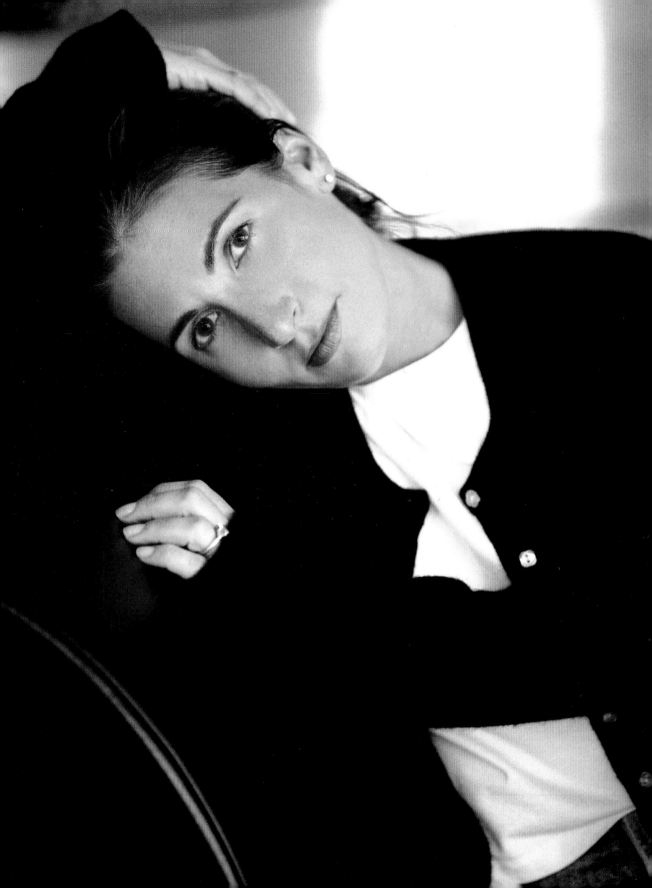

2

THE BOBBI BROWN PHILOSOPHY

I try to look my best, as most women do. I do it mainly for myself, but I like it when someone tells me I look pretty. I think everyone likes to hear that compliment; pretty is a magical word. After fifteen years as a professional makeup artist, having done thousands of women's faces, I believe looking pretty is not just about doing nice makeup or possessing exceptional God-given features. No, I am convinced that confidence is probably the most compelling element of real beauty. In every aspect of my life, I consciously strive to boost my self-confidence. I make a practice of limiting negativity and hassles that can drag me down or erode that self-assurance. A positive outlook shapes my roles at home and at work—as a wife and mother and as a makeup artist and the head of my own cosmetics company; it is, I hope, the guiding principle of this book.

PHILOSOPHY

What, exactly, is my beauty style? It is modern, pared-down, and realistic. It is makeup that is superwearable, long-lasting, and easy to apply. It is about a face that is pretty not because it is perfectly painted or artfully spackled but because it is smooth, natural, and healthy-looking. It is products that do not mask or disguise your own natural good looks, ethnicity, or skin tone. My beauty mission is to help women appreciate their own unique features, not those of a flawless supermodel or a breathtakingly beautiful actress. I want to enable every woman to develop her own beauty style.

My method of makeup application is straightforward and quite easy. I tend not to teach the most highly technical or intense applications since they can be time-consuming and produce looks that are outdated and overdramatic for everyday life. All of my methods are designed to be modulated—toned down or up—to your taste or to the occasion. That's because I feel that makeup should not be about rules—rather, it's about options.

Left: Makeup artist Bobbi Brown

My makeup palette is built around colors that are mistake-proof and classic enough to withstand the seasonal fluxes of fashion and beauty trends. All the shades in my makeup box have been specifically selected because they will endure—they will be current this month, this year, and five years from now. Period. There will be no rewriting of this book to reflect the next hot color off the runway or the next retro look in cosmetics to make a comeback. This is a guidebook that should help you look great forever.

A lot of women go in search of a makeup look. They get the steps written down for them on a piece of paper. Sometimes they'll even receive a diagram so that they may know where to put the makeup. They buy all the products and then go home, praying that they will be able to re-create the look themselves. If you think about it, does it make sense to do the same makeup every single day? The blush that looked fine on that September afternoon at the cosmetics counter when you bought all your new makeup may not do the trick on a February morning when you feel horrible and tired. Similarly, women go to skin specialists or to skin-care counters in department stores. They buy a lot of products, get a routine noted on paper, and go home to follow that routine morning and night. But will your skin need the same treatment on a ten-degree winter day as on a ninety-five-degree August day? Of course not.

I examine my face every day; it is my guide. I don't do the same makeup or the same skin care every day because neither the appearance of my skin nor the look of my face is exactly the same every day. It is much more useful and realistic to look at your face fresh every morning. Then you strive to do *that day* what is most beneficial and pretty *for you*.

My message is to learn to be your own skin-care expert and to learn to be your own makeup artist. It's not about owning one "miracle" cream or one "perfect" blush. It is about making the right choices based on your mood and look that day. Some days you may need a little bit of bronzing powder, while on others you may need a pop of soft pink. How and why you choose what you need that day will become second nature—and a whole lot more satisfying than following some unbending recipe.

It has long been my dream to do a comprehensive beauty book, in large part since so many women are in desperate need of the most basic beauty information so that they may feel confident to make their own makeup and skin-care decisions. Many women today face the double burden of having a career and maintaining a household, raising a family.

I am constantly trying to find the perfect balance between my work life and my home life. There never seems to be enough time.

For many of us there is an underlying pressure to look polished and presentable for work. Yet few of us have enough time to devote to our looks on a daily basis. That was my motivation for developing a streamlined system for the morning so you can apply your makeup quickly and get out the door fast, looking better than ever before. It is also my goal to help systematize and clean up your makeup kit so that it contains only the most basic items that you really love and actually use. You'll be surprised how much your life can be simplified just by pulling your makeup bag together.

I know from experience behind my own makeup counters that most women want to learn the fundamentals of makeup. Most women just want to look pretty. I never do a certain makeup look simply because it is this season's trend. I can honestly say that whenever I do makeup, I look at the woman carefully and consider her style and the constraints of her life. Is she a new mother? Is she laid-back? Is she a high-powered executive? Is she uncomfortable with some aspect of her face or making up?

My system is also adaptable to a changing daily schedule, and is flexible enough to work for the special occasions in your life and even bigger life changes. It is designed to address your worst beauty nightmare, those days when you feel that absolutely nothing will work. Next time you face an "ugly" day, you will know what to do. Chances are, you're doing too much!

My beauty philosophy is about creating a beauty style that works for you and is expressive of you. Trends come and go. Style endures.

It is much the same with fashion. Consider my most enduring clothing items: a great navy suit, a white T-shirt, the perfect (now seriously torn) blue jeans. I continue to love and wear these items because they are classic and always look good. That's my goal with makeup, too.

If you wear beautiful clothes but don't wear beautiful makeup, the clothes are somehow less beautiful. The total look is something less sophisticated. Perhaps there are times when that is exactly what you want. Sometimes if I feel my makeup is getting too serious, I rub some of it off and put on my motorcycle jacket. You have to balance the elements of your look. What you do on your face is related to the shoes you wear, your skirt length, and whether you're wearing a tailored jacket or a nubby cardigan. Style is about beauty *and* fashion and is communicated by what appears *above* and *below* your neck.

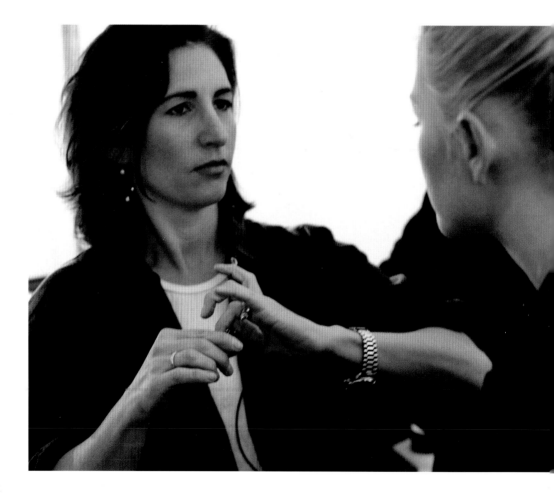

Keep it simple, real, and approachable. This is my mantra and my problem solver. This is the key to all my wardrobe dilemmas and the approach I take to my life, my makeup company, my work, my own face when I look in the mirror, and the makeup I apply to the thousands of real women and celebrities I work with every year. I am certain that I look my best when I enhance my own features, rather than masking or distorting them. I studied theatrical makeup (I have my bachelor's degree in it from Emerson College) and have the technical expertise to make a person look decades older or younger than she really is, to create scars or bruises, or to transform almost anyone into Marilyn Monroe or Claudia Schiffer. Yet I don't feel that such dramatic makeup measures serve us well in everyday life. I have developed a strong belief in a naturalistic approach to makeup. I have found that simple and natural makeup well applied always produces the most satisfying and beautiful results. It is also the most modern-looking and, ultimately, achievable.

Much of the "perfect" makeup you admire on faces in advertisements and magazines should probably come with the warning "Don't try this at home." To my taste, makeup that is retro, highly technical, stylized, and glamorized is not modern. Who has the time? Who has the energy? Who wants to look untouchable and painted?

That is not to say that I sometimes don't enjoy doing strong and creative makeup myself. Some people wrongly assume that I only do natural makeup. I welcome the opportunity to work on editorial photo shoots where I can create looks that are novel, completely unexpected, graphic, and artistic. I have done black-and-white lips, dark smoky eyes, shiny lips, greasy skin. No, these are not looks that are intended to be part our daily lifestyles. I wouldn't really recommend going out on a dinner date made up in this way. This sort of image serves another purpose altogether. It is about fantasy and dreaming. It is about stretching our imaginations and breaking down boundaries. If you are shocked by and attracted to an image of near-black lips, maybe you will be inspired to try wearing a deep berry- or a rich burgundy-colored lipstick.

What you *don't* know about images printed in magazines might surprise you. Sometimes models' faces are taped back at the hairline to create a

Bobbi at work, making up a model backstage at a fashion show.

more taut appearance and the more uplifted eyes of a starlet. Often eyebrows are dyed and plucked within a hair of extinction. What's more, the "perfect" face you might envy has probably been heavily doctored with the photographic process known as airbrushing or fixed to perfection in a computer. Real-life moles, dark circles, facial hair, pimples, enlarged pores, red splotches, bloodshot eyes, even saggy arms or thick thighs are all made to disappear. It is difficult to imagine that these same flawless actresses and models are women just like you. But I know very well from working with celebrities and models on photo shoots that they struggle with the same skin-care woes and makeup crises that you do. Believe me—*no one* is flawless and *no one* is immune from bad beauty days.

I've found that a lot of women feel insecure about the way they look. Helping women feel better about themsleves is a big motivation in doing the work I do in life. We can't help comparing ourselves to the perfected beauties we see on billboards, in magazines, and on television. Look, there's Cindy! Now there's Claudia! It's Christy! There's Elle! Each one is more gorgeous than the last. We know them by their first names. Supermodels have become our superstars. Somehow in the process, though, normal women are made to feel less than adequate and very unpretty.

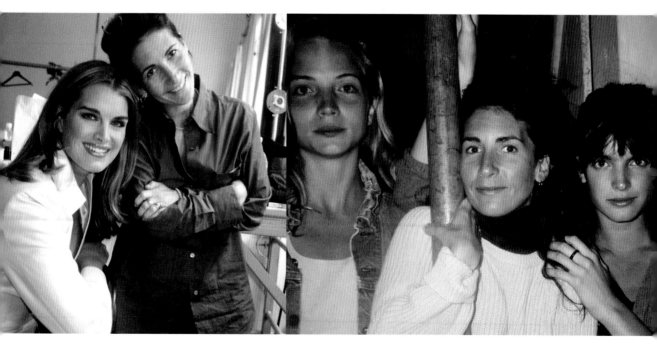

I grew up in a time when beauty was epitomized by tall, blond models who then would have been considered "all-American." Women like Cheryl Tiegs, Christie Brinkley, and Kelly Emberg defined beauty. Since I am five feet tall, with deep-set brown eyes, dark eyebrows, and brown hair, I didn't feel pretty. I often wonder how many thousands of other young women were (and probably still are) feeling inadequate because they do not conform to some narrow definition of pretty. Happily, models today are a much more diverse lot.

As I came into my own I realized the importance of being satisfied with the person that I am and the looks I was given. When I first started in the fashion business I sometimes felt inferior about my height. Now I've decided to make the most out of my small size—I rarely wear heels. Even more than appreciating who I am, I've learned to love myself for it.

The lesson I've learned in my career in the fashion world and what I

These pictures are from my own private photo journal. Here I am behind the scenes with some of my favorite subjects: (from far left) under the lights with Brooke Shields, on the road with Rachel Williams and Stephanie Seymour, a hug at the end of the day from Jennifer Beals, a height comparison with Niki Taylor.

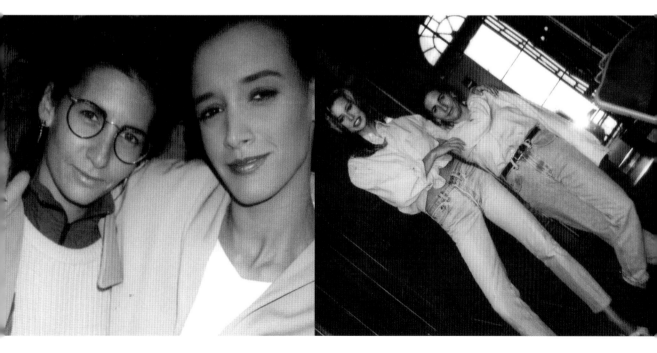

most wish to communicate through my makeup is to love the features that make you special. In talking to women about makeup and their looks, I often feel as if I am part makeup artist and part therapist, helping women see and appreciate the special qualities about themselves. That really isn't so surprising given that our looks are so closely tied to our identity as a person.

Through years of observation I have noticed that beauty has as much to do with your own features and makeup expertise as your self-image. It's really so simple: Women who have confidence are more beautiful. Think about the confidence exuded by women like Anjelica Huston, Diane Sawyer, Jodie Foster, and Annette Bening. It is their strength of character, as much as their looks, that gives them their unmistakable presence.

In my work, I prefer doing makeup on "imperfect" beauties—women who do not possess the most standard, conventional features. It's much more interesting for me as a makeup artist. I recently was asked to do a story for *Harper's Bazaar*: Create a signature makeup look, on a model of my choice, that epitomizes modern good looks. I chose Jaime Rishar precisely because her look is a little off. She isn't model-tall (in fact, she is tiny), and she is extremely pale and not classically featured. I like

Two of my favorite faces: Christie Brinkley (left) and Phoebe Cates.

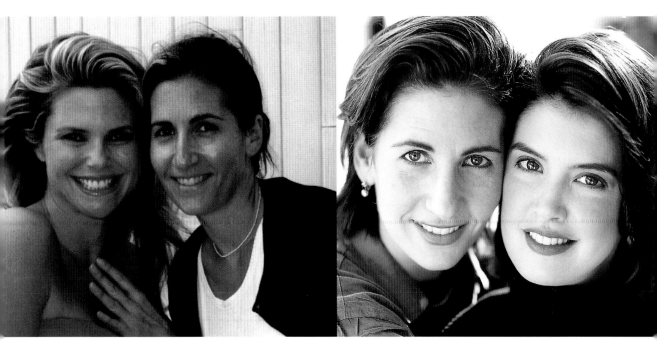

that she is not a typical "cookie-cutter" beauty. I also like that she is real: She comes from a real town, has a real family, uses her own, real name,and is down-to-earth. Her wit and sense of humor come through in her eyes and the way she holds her face. She doesn't have a vacant stare. That, to me, is modern beauty.

More than anything, I hope this book will help break down some of our culture's definitions of "perfect" beauty and "classic" features. I would love to abolish the notion that a makeover will somehow make you into a better person. I prefer the term makeunder, in the sense that only in paring down makeup do you reach a look that best allows your personality to shine through.

Every woman has some feature that she can highlight and make the most of—a strong nose, prominent eyebrows, full lips, deep-set eyes, or a pronounced hair color, like blue-black or bright red. The very same characteristics women don't like about themselves are often the ones I feel makes them special and beautiful. Jodie Foster is not a classic beauty. Nor is Demi Moore. Neither of them has a typical Hollywood or Madison Avenue look, the small nose, full lips, big, blue eyes, blond hair, and tall stature that epitomizes beauty on billboards and in films. But to my eye, both of these women are modern and far more interesting than a conventional notion of perfection. In the end, the ideal we should all strive for is a very personal definition of our own beauty. How better to achieve a look that is unmatchable, perfectly attainable, and utterly unique than to be your own true self?

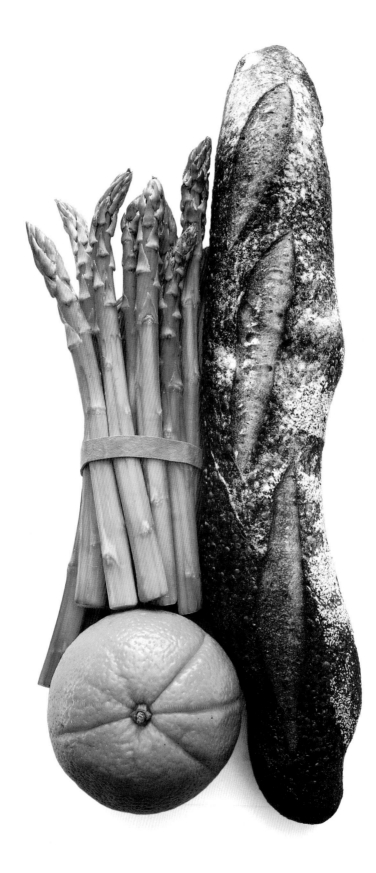

3

BODY BASICS: DIET AND EXERCISE

Through my work as a professional makeup artist, I see and speak with thousands of women every year. What I hear is often striking and disturbing. Lots of women tell me that they hate the way they look. Many tell me of their deep desire to be prettier, skinnier, taller, younger, or sexier. Their language is strong and sometimes even self-abusive.

It is obvious to me that the majority of women I come in contact with are not content with their looks. A large number are obsessed with their bodies and their faces—sometimes caring so much that it becomes an unhealthy negative emotion. My crusade is to make women comfortable in their skin. Looking good really does comes from within—from feeling good about yourself.

There are certain basic things about yourself that you must accept, such as your height and your body's frame. There are other things, however, that you can take control of and change. I was not born tall and skinny. So instead of trying to be what I am not, I center my energies on feeling good with my frame. I always try to focus on the positive—like the aspects of my body over which I have control: eating as healthfully as possible and being as fit and strong as possible. My message is: Take control of what you can; then you will be your most beautiful.

DIET

If I eat well, I look good. If I don't, well, my looks definitely suffer. It seems almost old-fashioned to talk about the connection between healthful eating and good looks, but that link is fundamental.

I don't believe in fad diets like the grapefruit diet or powdered-drink diets, or whatever is this moment's fad solution. The truth is that I do not believe in the concept of dieting at all. I think that dieting is based on denial, which you will ultimately resent and rebel against. You are destined to fail. Instead, if you partake in a good healthful diet for life, an eating plan based on a diet rich in whole grains, vegetables and fruits, and low-fat proteins—you are destined for long-term success.

We should all be realistic in our expectations, not fanatical. When you are on the go with lots of commitments, you are not going to have time to cook low-fat, healthful meals. Make sure that when you grab something to eat from the refrigerator, you have healthful options like yogurt, fruit, or vegetables. When I am out and about, I make sure I have good, healthful snacks tucked away in my bag—an apple, a Power Bar, or whole-grain crackers—for the times when I am suddenly starving.

When you eat things that are not ideal (and we all do), make sure it's worth it. It's not about grabbing a candy bar every afternoon at 4 P.M. Rather, order a dessert one night when you are out for dinner and savor it! Then, the next day, instead of dwelling on it or letting it trigger a week of out-of-control eating, just get on with your normal, healthful routine. Don't be too hard on yourself for an indulgence every now and then. It might sound clichéd, but I view every day as another opportunity to eat as healthfully as possible.

I am a big believer in whole natural foods. I read labels carefully and try to avoid food with lots of additives and chemicals. For that reason, I tend to buy most of my food in a health-food store. The cookies I buy for my kids contain no sugar, no dyes, and no preservatives. It costs a little more, but it's worth it to me in the long run.

Drinking a lot of water also works for me, both by staving off my appetite (often when you think you are hungry, you are really just thirsty!) and giving my skin a clearer, plumped-up appearance. Water also keeps me going when I exercise, by keeping me hydrated, which in turn gives me energy. I find that by squirting lemon in water I drink more—and enjoy it a lot more.

EXERCISE

Exercise gives me more than a toned, strong body. If I am feeling down, exercise lifts my mood. If I am feeling tired, it gives me energy that I've found to be truly addictive. I also find that good, consistent exercise makes me more realistic and accepting of things I don't like about myself. It is as much for my mind as for my body.

I try to exercise at least five times a week. That can mean walking for fifteen minutes, or it can mean a serious, ninety-minute aerobics class. I make it a point to vary what I do so I don't get bored. We all have good

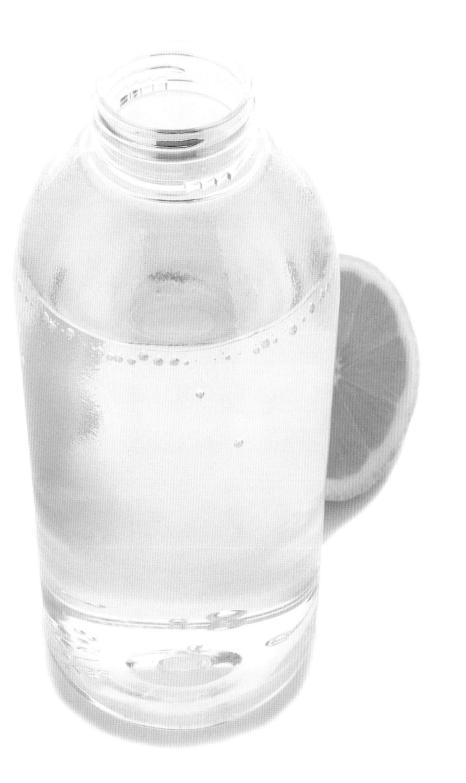

excuses for why we don't exercise. In my life, I have attempted to face all my excuses and find solutions by creating different fitness options for different situations. If it's a choice between spending time on my body or spending time with my children, I use my baby jogger and no one loses out. If being strong and fit is a priority in your life, no matter how busy you are, you can find time for it.

Gyms: Find a stretching, toning, yoga, or aerobics class at a gym. Vary the kind of class that you take to keep yourself interested. The very presence of other students will motivate you. (Kids are not an excuse. If you have small children, find a gym that has child care or baby-sitting.)

If you use machines, vary your workout by switching aerobics machines, or try doing a circuit, i.e., eight to ten minutes each on three or more types of machines that require different kinds of movement (treadmill, bicycle, cross-country ski machine, and StairMaster, say). The time flies, and it's a lot more fun. Below are, some of my favorite exercise options.

Walking/Running: Walking and running are by far the most convenient forms of exercise. Try varying distances and routes to keep yourself interested. If you have a hard time getting out of bed in the morning, set out your complete workout outfit—from athletic shoes to cap—the night before. I find that the hardest part is sometimes just getting dressed. Once I do that, I will definitely do the workout.

If you live in a cold (or extremely warm) climate, you might explore indoor walking at your local mall. Many malls even have walking clubs and open their doors early for the convenience of the walkers.

Jumping Rope: Jumping rope is an amazing aerobic activity. Try to keep movement controlled and small—like a boxer would jump rope. Work up to 100 jumps. (Be sure to stretch your calves afterward.)

Doing the Stairs: Going up and down my home stairs (two at a time) ten to twenty times is great exercise. You can also use the stairwell in your apartment building or gym.

Personal Trainers: Having a trainer come to your home effectively eliminates most exercise excuses. If you can afford this option, interview several trainers to find one you really like. Or, on a one-shot basis, ask a trainer to create an exercise program tailored for you and your lifestyle.

Videos: A great at-home exercise option. Doing the same tape again and again wouldn't work for me, so I try to vary their content. Choices include aerobic dance, weight training, yoga, and stretching.

Weight Training: Be sure that weight-bearing movement is a part of your exercise routine. Doing a series of exercises with light hand weights will define muscles (it will not bulk you up as so many women fear). It can improve your posture and help build bone density, which, in turn, prevents osteoporosis.

Fitness Fallacies

• Abdominal exercises can help tone your stomach—but they will *not flatten it.* Increase aerobic exercise and reduce fat in your diet to work away fat from your body.

• Lifting weights will not create body-builder muscles . . . but if you are worried about bulking up, do higher repetitions with lower weights (even two-pound weights work).

• Stretching cold muscles *before* working out is a bad idea—and can

Below is Jody Jarel, the woman who always inspires me to go just a little bit further than I think myself capable. (Just look at her perfect body!) Jody teaches the most amazing aerobics classes, and sometimes comes to my home to train me one-on-one. She is a source of energy and inspiration.

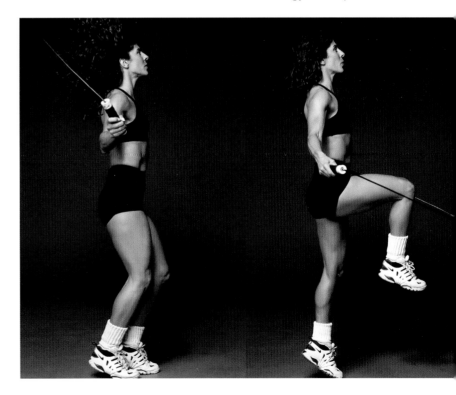

even be injurious. It is a good idea to warm the body up for a few minutes doing leg lifts, a brisk walk, or a light jog before doing any kind of stretching that will, in turn, help prevent injury during your fitness activity. Stretch again at the end of your workout to prevent soreness the next day.

• "No pain, no gain" is bad fitness thinking. I believe, on the other hand, that *if you truly like the activity* you are engaged in, you are more apt to stick to it and see real gains. Stretching properly helps reduce injury as well as aches and pains.

On-the-Road Exercise

If I am traveling, I stay only at hotels with gyms. And these days so many hotels have added fitness facilities, it's never a problem. Call ahead to be sure.

Fitness Vacations

I live in a house with boys (I'm including my husband in this category!), so our vacations often center around sports: hiking, skiing, horseback riding. Even though I am not a natural-born athlete, I love doing sporting activities together as a family. Anyone can be a born-again athlete. If there is an activity you are interested in, what better way to learn than to take a vacation doing it!

BODY BASICS

Massage: I consider the occasional massage a basic necessity, not a selfish expense or luxury. I find that my body truly needs the muscle therapy, given all the travel and exercise that I do. Afterward, I look flushed in such a pretty way, and I am so very calm. The oils used are extremely nourishing for the skin.

If you don't know a masseuse or masseur, ask at your local Y or skin-care salon. Or go to a massage center, like Great American Backrub, for quicker, clothes-on head, neck, foot, and shoulder treatments.

Since so many of us have a hard time paying for the luxury of our own massage, consider giving gift certificates for a massage to your friends or family for birthdays or on a special occasion.

Body Polishing: One of my best body experiences was a salt rub I had at a spa many years ago. It left my entire body soft and smooth—I felt like a new person.

To make your own salt rub, mix the coarsest salt you can find with a little gentle liquid soap. (Dr. Bronner's peppermint is my favorite soap.)

Using your hands or a loofah mitt, suds the mixture all over your body in the shower (scrub extra hard on your elbows, heels, and knees). Rinse thoroughly. Pat your body dry and rub a rich cream or oil all over. Do not use a cream containing alpha hydroxy acids after a scrub; your skin is too sensitive, and it would sting.

Cellulite Creams/Remedies: We all wish they would work, but they don't. Unfortunately, there are no such miracles out there, so creams and treatments that claim to treat cellulite are just a waste of money.

If you have a body part that you obsess over, pamper that area—exfoliate it regularly and apply rich creams to improve your skin's texture. Accept it, own it, and move on to things you can do something about.

Shaving: Shaving your legs and underarms isn't a chore if you get in the habit of doing it every day or every other day in the shower. Use some kind of lubricant or risk chafing your skin. Classic men's shaving creams work well. If you're ever caught without shaving cream, remember that hair conditioner works well.

Waxing: Some women wax their legs and swear by the results: a perfectly smooth, hairless surface. But since I cannot bear growing my leg hair the ten days to two weeks that is necessary before doing a full leg wax, I will never know. I do recommend waxing other areas, however: The bikini line and upper lip are the two most common waxing zones. You may choose to go to a salon or to do it yourself, as follows:

Heat wax (I like No Tweeze brand, which is sold at beauty supply stores), but don't allow it to get too hot. Dust nontalcum baby powder over the area first; then, using a smooth wooden stick, smooth wax over the area. Allow wax to dry a bit, but not completely. Remove it quickly and smoothly. First you peel back a corner, then rip the rest away. Afterward, apply soothing cream on top.

Note: Do not wax during or just before your period, as it's more painful—skin can be extremely sensitive.

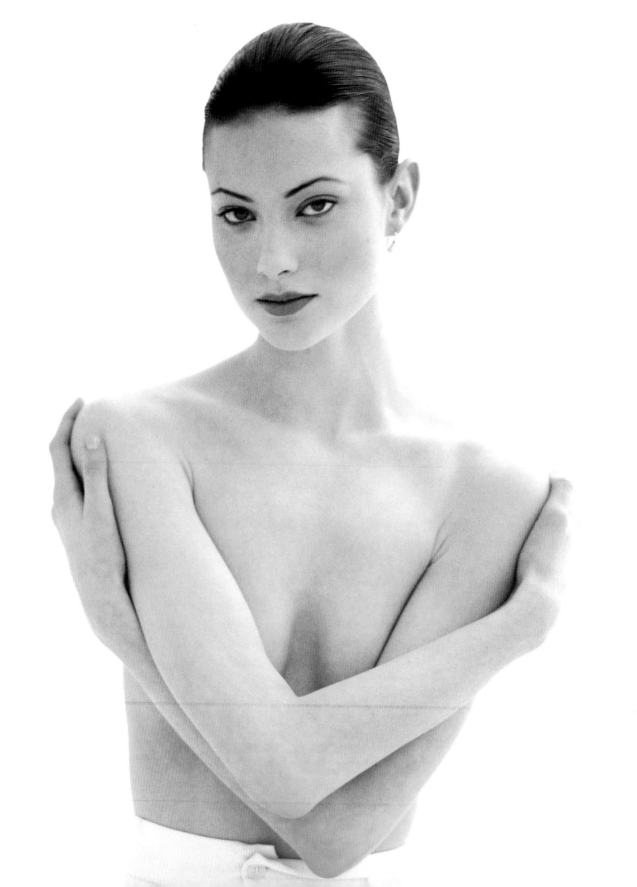

4

SKIN BASICS

Perfectly smooth, flawless skin: It is the most highly desired element of beauty, but, for many, the most elusive. If you were born with and have maintained lovely skin, consider yourself lucky. For the rest of us, though, the quest for a good complexion often proves frustrating, as so much of what affects our skin is completely out of our control. Genetics plays a big part. No potions or lotions will ever change the basic genetic makeup of your skin. Your skin's allergies and its sensitivities to ingredients and pollution is something you can react to but not easily alter. Stress is another detrimental factor. Yes, we'd all like less of it, but it is part of all of our lives. Stress can have the effect of overdrying already dry skin and triggering breakouts in oily or difficult skin.

I believe in taking charge of the skin-care issues over which you do have control. Good skin is clearly not just about what you put on your skin but how you conduct your life. I see a giant difference in my face when I am rested and relaxed. Getting adequate sleep helps one deal with stress. Drinking plenty of water and doing physical activities help contribute to a clearer, smoother complexion. (This is one of the reasons I try to exercise at least five times a week—see chapter 3.) And I can see a definite difference in my face on the days I get to class or do a half hour on the StairMaster. Now, a few things *not* to do . . .

Smoking, besides its grave medical consequences, is one of the worst things you can do for your face. A regular smoking habit in your twenties and thirties can age your skin by as much as ten to fifteen years, but may only become visible in your forties. The pursing lip action you apply on cigarettes will result in permanent lip lines all around your mouth. Skin takes on an unattractive yellowish cast, and dark circles become more prominent. Working as a makeup artist backstage at the fashion shows and on photography shoots, I exist in a world of smokers. Models smoke because they hope it will help them stay thin and look cool—and because they are bored: There is so much downtime in this business. Thankfully, even when I was younger, I was never seduced by the so-called glamour of cigarettes. I am pretty militant in asking people not to smoke around me or my kids.

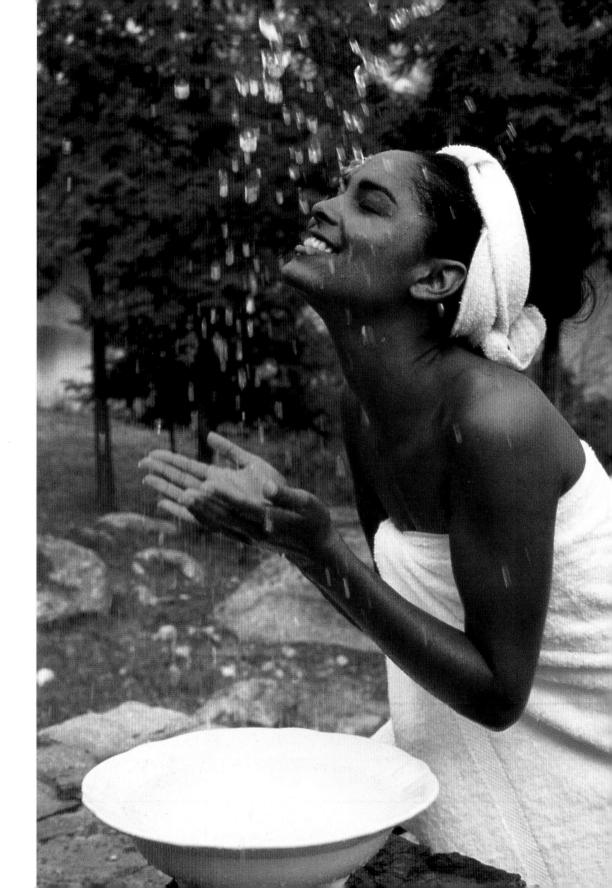

So think ahead. Be aware that smoking ages your face measurably. It will rob you of your youthful good looks before you are ready to give them up.

Sun exposure is equally, if not more, harmful to your skin. If you limit exposure to the sun and are careful to wear high-SPF sunblock as well as protective clothing, sunglasses, and a hat, you are, in effect, preventing future lines and wrinkles and, quite possibly, skin cancer.

As scientists learn more and more about the sun's rays, sun-protection products will probably become more sophisticated. We do know that the sun's long UVA rays are the aging rays, since they go deep into the skin, destroying its support structure of collagen and elastin. The short UVB rays are cancer-causing, and infrared rays are the heat penetrators, which can feel good, but are also responsible for serious damage. Look for the most state-of-the-art sunblocks, which protect from all three types of rays.

Note: Tanning salons are unregulated in this country. Despite claims of safety, tanning beds can be extremely harmful.

CLEANSING

A lot of women in their thirties and forties continue to use bar soap to cleanse their faces. I think soap is the worst thing in the world for your skin. Others use soapy cleansers, some of which are strong enough to clean the dishes. Perhaps our tendency to overcleanse is based on the fact that most of us began a regular cleansing routine when we were in our teens or early twenties, when our skin was at its oiliest. Women of all ages should be concerned about cleansing their skin, not stripping it. We all should be aware that our skin changes, depending on the season, the climate we're in, travel, etc. And our skin changes with time. Even if you had oily skin in your teens, it's quite possible that your skin is only partly oily or normal later on.

TAKING CHARGE

My advice is to learn to be your own skin-care expert. It is important to look at your own face in the mirror and see for yourself what's going on.

The idea is not to have just one product or just one daily routine for skin care. It's best to have options at your fingertips for whatever you may face in the mirror. In the summer, your skin may be drier on the surface, thanks to air-conditioning, but oilier underneath. When pregnant, your skin may become much drier or much oilier. Around the holidays, your skin may act oilier. In the coldest months of the winter, your skin may well be drier. If you've traveled a lot by plane, chances are that—no matter your normal skin type—your skin is probably suddenly behaving like dry skin.

Sometimes I use a cream with AHAs (alpha hydroxy acids) for my skin—and sometimes I don't. When my skin feels dry, I layer an AHA lotion with a richer face cream on top. If my skin is extremely dry, I'll put on a beeswax protective barrier, but that's something I wouldn't do every day. For me, it's not about switching around products or routine. Rather, it's about always having the right choices at my fingertips.

Another key to developing the right skin-care program for yourself is not to go in search of a fountain of youth. Do not be pulled in by promises of younger-looking skin. Don't rush to your nearest department store to buy this week's newest "miracle" cream. Instead, seek to find a flexible routine that makes your skin healthy, smooth, and clear. That should be your main mission.

The following is a menu of the range of products each woman should keep at home and have available the moment she needs it.

Skin-Care Necessities

gel cleanser: gentle, nonstripping formula for oily skin or, in hot weather, for all skin types

creamy cleanser: choose one that rinses off with water

AHA lotion or cream: two intensities (not recommended for extremely sensitive skin)

rich facial cream: use only if AHAs are not moisturizing enough

oil-free lotion: for oily skin

nonoily eye makeup remover

eye cream

body lotion

pumice stone: keep in shower to smooth rough spots and calluses on feet

Skin-Care Extras

toner: nonalcohol formula; often sold as a must-use step, toners are truly optional

gentle, grainy scrub: for days when you really need to exfoliate (skip if you have sensitive skin); helps clear blackheads

soothing mask: look for hydrating, creamy formulas. Cucumber is a natural soother, as is calendula. Use to calm the face when especially tired or after sun or wind exposure.

clay mask: for oily, acne-prone skin, or for all skin types for deep cleansing in the summer

dry oil spray for body: may be applied in the shower

loofah or body brush: keep in shower to exfoliate arms, legs, elbows, knees, and thighs

balm or heavy cream protectant: for lips, cuticles, and face (in extreme cold or dry conditions)

Then, depending on how your skin is behaving (oily or normal-to-dry), you'll need the following basic products.

Oily Skin

Cleanser: Use a gentle gel formula. Rinse away carefully, counting at least ten splashes. (If it's winter or if you have been spending time on airplanes, your skin may be behaving more like normal-to-dry skin, in which case you should use a creamy cleanser.)

Toner: Avoid toners containing alcohol, as they can dry the surface of your skin, blocking impurities beneath the surface. Overdrying the skin is one of the biggest mistakes women with oily skin make. Toners containing AHAs work well to help smooth skin's texture. Cucumber water is another nice option. Use a clean cotton pad.

Moisturizer: Use a gel, an oil-free moisturizer, or a mattifying cream specially made for oily skin (it dries matte on the skin and minimizes large pores and smoothes surface texture imperfections). If you are drier around the eye area (most people are), apply a richer cream to that area at night.

Foundation: Use oil-free formulas.

Exfoliant: Use a gentle, grainy scrub twice weekly, concentrating on blackhead-prone areas like the nose and chin.

Special Care: Clay mask.

Normal-to-Dry Skin

Cleanser: Use a creamy cleanser that rinses off with water. I don't advise using a tissue-off cleansing cream, as they can leave a residue. You may consider using a gel cleanser once a week for a more thorough cleansing, or switch to the gel cleanser in hot, humid weather.

Toner: If you like using a toner, choose an extremely gentle formula (like rosewater) on a clean cotton pad to prime your skin for the moisturizer. If your cleanser rinses off well, skip the toner. (Or, if you choose, use toner in summer.)

Moisturizer: Make sure your moisturizer is rich but absorbs completely into your skin. If your skin feels taut five minutes after application, either the moisturizer formula is not rich enough or it has been too sparingly applied. At night, use heavier moisturizing cream. If you have especially dry spots, use an AHA lotion all over your face and richer hydrating cream on those dry areas. Remember, you don't have to treat your whole face in the same way.

Foundation: Use a rich, creamy formula. Oil-free foundation or tinted moisturizer is a summer option, but be sure to use a light facial lotion first.

Exfoliant: Use creamy, gentle AHAs, but only if your skin does not become red or irritated.

Special Care: Hydrating mask.

Note: Do not use clay masks if your skin is severely dry.

ALPHA HYDROXY ACIDS (AHAS)

This is a term used to denote one of the many naturally occurring components of milk (lactic acid), sugarcane (glycol acid), and apples (malic acid), among others. The smoothing benefit of these acids is legendary: Cleopatra, for one, was famous for her milk baths. In recent years these acids have been refined, concentrated, and added to an increasingly large number of products, such as body lotions, face creams, cuticle creams, toners, self-tanners, etc. Today's AHAs work on a molecular level to exfoliate or turn over your skin so that it is softer and smoother on the surface. AHAs eliminate the flaking or redness or sensitivity associated with manual exfoliation (grainy scrubs) and lead to visibly smoother skin. AHAs are as close to a skin-care miracle as I have ever found, and, I would venture to say, they are here to stay.

For me, AHAs are for skin care what fluoride was for dental health. I am a big fan; they help me get my skin as smooth-looking as I like.

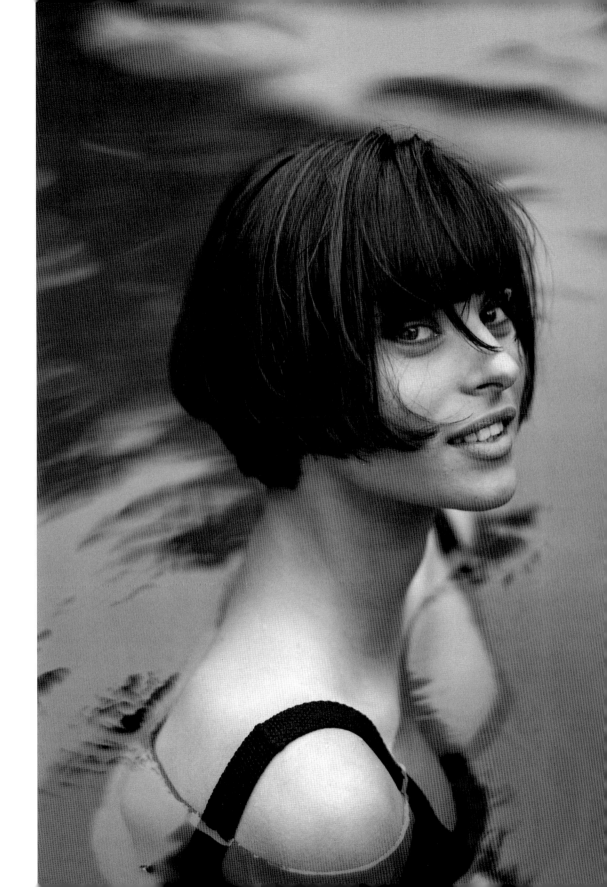

Nonetheless, let your skin be the judge. If you experience redness or sting-ing while using any product containing AHAs, cease using it. While some companies disclose the percentage of AHAs in a given product (i.e., 2 percent, 4 percent), that number can be confusing; other ingredients may counteract the active AHAs. My advice is to start with a gentle formula every other day and watch how your skin reacts.

AHAs can be used by all skin types. They can be especially good in combating blackheads, dehydrated skin, and an unevenness in the skin's texture.

FACIALS

There is no national standard and no licensing bureau for facialists in this country, so every facial has the potential to be a brave new experience. Nor is there any universally acknowledged beauty benefit to having regular facials. It's one of those things that you should judge for yourself.

The salon world has its own language and the list of services at any local salon can be daunting in itself:

glycolic acid facial: a favorite of mine, this is usually a strong exfoliating session

hydrating facial: gooey and creamy, great if you have been traveling a lot

deep-cleansing facial: good for cleaning out blackheads, if you don't mind having the facialist pressing and squeezing the impurities from your face. Normally, the face is steamed, manually cleaned, then soothed with a mask.

lymphatic drainage facial: meant to activate your body's own toxin-fighting systems

I go for facials only about twice a year because I like the relaxing and de-stressing effect it has on me. There are moments when I feel I need an intense deep-cleansing treatment.

More important than the type of facial you opt for, though, is the facialist herself. Do not walk in for a salon facial without an appointment. Talk to someone who gets facials regularly—although you should keep in mind that one woman's dream facial is another woman's nightmare. Call a salon and speak to the facialist before booking a time. You will want to know that the person is well trained. Inquire where she received training and if she has some sort of training certificate. A certificate is not required by law but may be an indication of her level of expertise. Ask how long she has been at it. A few weeks or months is not long enough. Does she also do manicures and pedicures? The best facialists will have no time for anything else. Ask what the format of the facial is—how long it will take, what products are used, etc. What you *don't* want is a facialist who puts a mask on your face and then disappears for twenty minutes.

My favorite kind of facial is soothing and healing. I like a facialist whose hands do not leave me for the entire session. While my mask is on, she might do a gentle neck and shoulder massage or a moisturizing massage for my hands or feet.

BODY CARE

Given how much time we spend obsessing about our faces and how much money on products for our faces, it seems strange that the face is such a small percentage of our body's total surface area. Moisturizing every reachable inch of your body after a shower should be as automatic as brushing your teeth. I like to rub oil into my skin when I am in the shower—it hydrates my dry skin and saves me time when I get out. (Pat skin dry with a towel so as not to rub off the oil.)

Feet are the most neglected part of a woman's body. I recommend keeping a pumice stone in the shower so that smoothing away calluses and dry skin on the heels and pads of your feet becomes part of your shower routine. Use the pumice on the rough edges of your toes and on thick fingernail cuticles—be gentle, though. You can use the same rich balm you use on your lips for your heels and toes. It makes a good cuticle moisturizer for fingernails, too.

DERMATOLOGISTS

When should you go to a dermatologist? When things get serious and you can't handle a skin-care problem on your own. Don't waste your time and money seeking instant cures at the skin-care counter at a department store. Below are some of the most common reasons for seeking medical advice.

Acne: By my definition, acne is constantly present blemishes, more than an occasional or monthly breakout. If you have acne, seek the care of a dermatologist. The range of options today—from topical antibiotics to oral antibiotics—pretty much guarantees that no one should have to suffer from serious acne.

Note: If you are taking birth control pills, let your dermatologist know the exact name of your medication. Certain pills will make you more acne-prone. Others can even help those who suffer from breakouts. Dermatologists do not always inquire about this, so bring the subject up yourself.

Allergic Reactions: If you experience redness or itching, hives or blotches, you should stop using all but the most gentle cleansing products and go see a dermatologist. It would be useful to think in advance about what might be the problem. Consider if you have started using a new product or if there is some new aspect to your daily routine—a new laundry detergent, toothpaste, skin cream, mascara, or shade of eye shadow could be the cause of your reaction. If you suspect something particular, bring along the product (or its ingredient label) to show your doctor.

Question: Is it better *not* to wear makeup when I have blemishes? Won't makeup make my breakouts worse?

Answer: Wearing makeup will not negatively affect your skin's condition as long as you cleanse your face thoroughly at night. In fact, I recommend wearing some coverage so that your skin looks better and you feel better about it. The dermatologists who recommend not wearing makeup are usually men.

- Use a creamy-textured, tinted, oil-free moisturizer or an oil-free foundation to create a smooth texture so that there will be no clumping on blemishes.
- Use your foundation shade (not your concealer) with the concealer brush to cover pimples.
- Avoid overdrying products that will roughen your skin's texture.

    Remember: Drying the skin's surface will simply block impurities and prevent them from exiting on their own.
- While moisturizing might seem counterintuitive with troubled skin, the very products you might use for blemishes can cause surface dryness. Besides, moisturizer will create a smoother appearance and allow makeup to set better.

SUN CARE

Given all that we know about the dangers of the sun, there is no other option than to make a practice of wearing sunscreen. Medically, there is the risk—ever increasing—of skin cancer. Cosmetically, we know that unprotected exposure to the sun will lead to brown spots, premature wrinkling, and a tough, leathery texture to the skin. A recent study I read shows that even a few minutes spent in intense sun without proper protection will result in measurable damage to the skin. The reality is that we all enjoy time in the sun—swimming, gardening, and playing out-of-doors with our kids. My advice is simply to be smart about it.

Since having children, I've learned how very treacherous the sun can be. I am constantly applying waterproof, high-SPF sunblock to my children's skin. Parents who do not protect their kids' skin and like the tanned look on babies and toddlers are really doing their children a grave disservice.

Sun Block Use: SPF 8 is sufficient for daily wear—going out on errands, on your way to work, out for a walk at lunchtime—any outdoor exposure that is limited to twenty minutes or less. To make life easier, choose a daytime

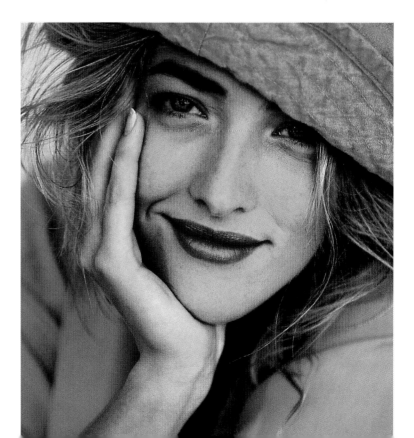

moisturizer that contains sunscreen. I don't recommend foundations containing sunscreens, as smooth texture is usually compromised.

Makeup and Sunblock: If you have limited exposure to the sun, wear a moisturizer containing sunblock (SPF 8 to 15) and then wear your make-up as usual. If you are outside for longer periods of time (playing golf or tennis, say), concentrate on proper sun protection and save the makeup for later. The highest protection and waterproof sunblocks do not work well under makeup, as they tend to make the face sticky and moist.

Chemical v. Nonchemical Blocks: Nonchemical sun products are the most foolproof and effective, and tend not to aggravate even the most sensitive skin. They contain titanium dioxide, whose microparticles actually block sun from harming skin. The drawback to these products is that they have a white or pasty appearance.

Chemical sunblocks protect skin thanks to sun-protective ingredients contained in the emulsion. Some people have allergies to components of chemical sunblocks (PABA is one common culprit). Waterproof formulas tend to be the most sensitizing.

Exposure Time: When you know that you will be outside for more than a few minutes, use an SPF 15 or higher. The truth is, you will still get some color with high protection. If you will be on the beach, playing golf or tennis, or gardening, try to remember to apply your sunblock at home at least one half hour before beginning your activity to allow the product to absorb. Apply a generous amount of sun protection. (The SPF number is based on a surprisingly generous slathering of sunblock.)

Be careful to avoid the eye area when applying sunblock, especially when using waterproof formulas, which can sting and make eyes tear. Reapply sun protection after swimming (especially if formula is not waterproof) and after more than two hours in the sun.

Sun-protection products should be discarded after one year, because their active ingredients will begin to lose their protective powers. Remember to apply an ample amount for full protection and don't forget your lips and under your eyes—two spots on the body where skin is extremely thin and more prone to burning.

Wear a hat and sunglasses whenever you are out in the sun: I never go outside in the summer without my baseball cap and shades.

TAKING IT OFF

Before washing your face in the evening, I recommend using a nonoily formula of eye makeup remover on a clean cotton pad to wipe away mascara, liner, and shadow. Nonoily removers (i.e., gel or liquid formulas) are important for several reasons. Oily removers can aggravate eyes. They can also can cause makeup to travel over your face so that it becomes very difficult to wash off. (If you wake up in the morning with mascara smeared on your face, oily eye makeup remover may be at fault.) Also, by using a nonoily remover, you have the option of reapplying makeup should you plan to go out later on; makeup will not take over an oil formula remover.

Nonoily makeup remover also lifts lipstick off completely and can be used to clean your lip brush. It has also helped me avert disaster more than once by lifting makeup stains from my clothing.

After taking off eye makeup and lip color, use cleansing cream or gel to remove all foundation, concealer, and powder. If you have bangs or if your hair falls into your face, use a headband or an elastic to pull back your hair so that you are sure to clean your face at the hairline.

Tip: After washing face, dip a Q-tip into nonoily remover and run it gently over your eyelashes to remove any residual mascara.

Oil-Based Makeup

If you are in theater and wear oil-based makeup for performances—or if you simply prefer a heavy base—good old-fashioned cold cream is the best remover. (It's also a good thing to keep around the house for removing the kids' makeup at Halloween!)

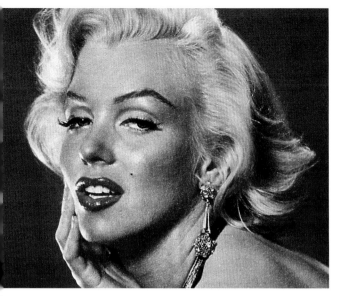
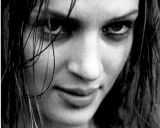
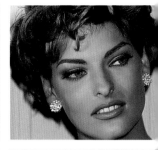
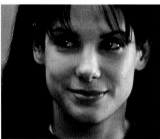
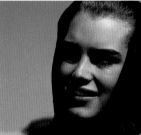
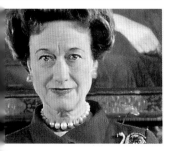
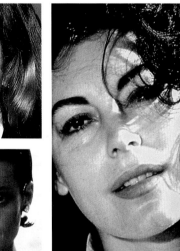
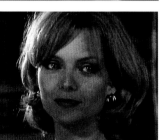
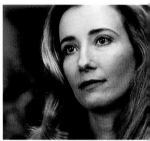
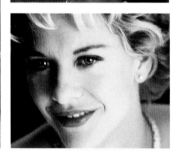
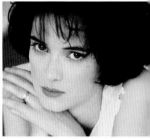
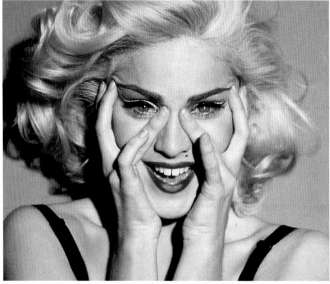
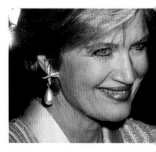
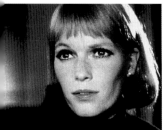
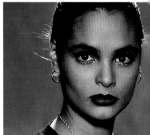

5

"IMPERFECT" BEAUTY: TAKING A "FLAW" AND MAKING IT YOUR MOST STRIKING FEATURE

I love a cleft in a woman's chin. I love really pale skin. I love deep-set eyes, extremely full lips, and strong, hooked noses. For me, it's not "Oh, how do I fix it?" Rather, it's claiming the features that make you who you are and making the most of them. Some call these qualities "flaws," but I find that they are the key to finding one's own beauty identity.

My definition of perfect beauty is that it be unique and completely individual. Unfortunately, my way of thinking is not yet universally accepted. No one ever told me as a child that my deep-set eyes were beautiful—but I now know that they are a striking element of my look. No one ever says that freckles are nice—but I think they are beautiful and should never be hidden.

It happens all the time: The very feature women complain to me about is precisely what I find most beautiful. And it's no wonder women don't like these features, since most of us have never heard them complimented. In a perfect world, mothers would remind their daughters each morning how beautiful their strong noses are, how lovely their deep-set brown eyes or pale skin, and how special their curly red hair or full lips. In a perfect world, we would grow up to accept ourselves for our special traits and to be genuinely content with our natural looks. We would possess an endless amount of self-confidence.

But too often this is not the case. Mothers, themselves feeling insecure about a particular feature, pass that feature on to their daughters along with a sense of shame or insufficiency about it. Boyfriends or husbands pick up on a woman's feelings of inadequacy, sometimes making her feel even worse. It is an unhappy cycle.

I refuse to accept that the only perfect beauty is that of a Barbie doll or a supermodel. Instead, I find beauty in the flaws, those characteristics that don't fit society's narrow definition of beauty. Sadly, women who have these characteristics have been taught not to like them. The challenge is to reverse this way of thinking.

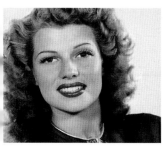
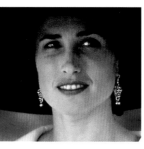
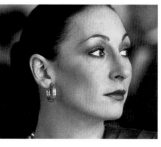
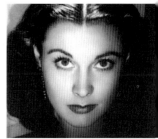
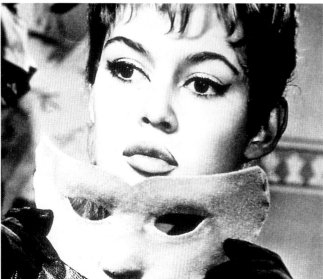
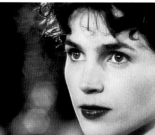
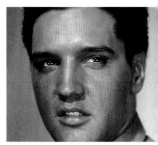
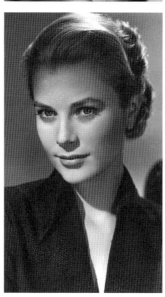
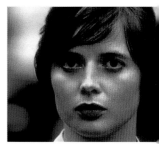
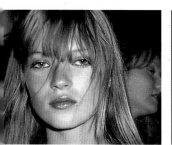
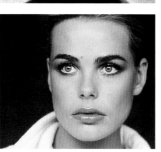
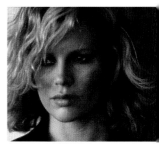
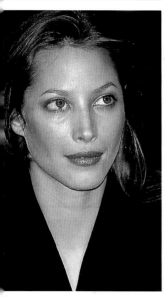
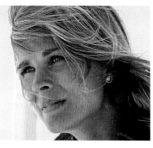
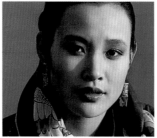
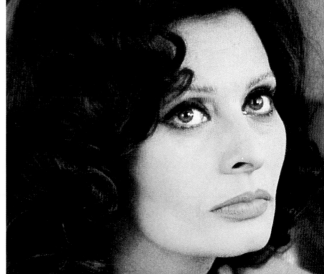

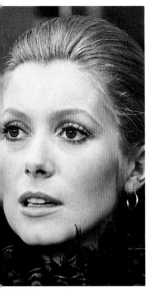
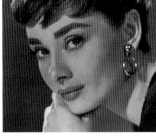
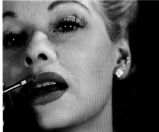
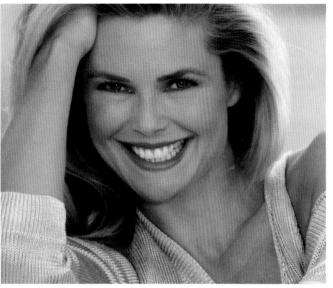
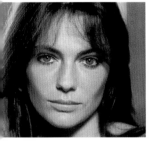
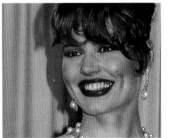
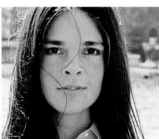
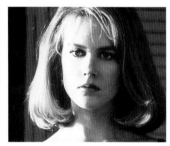
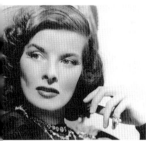
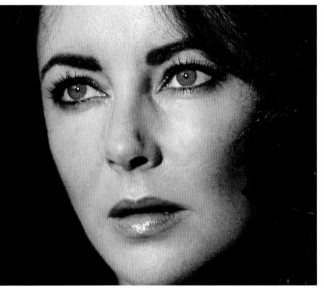
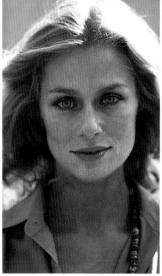
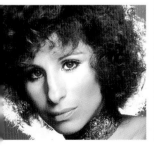
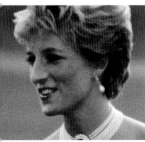
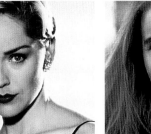
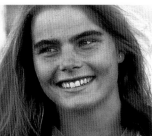
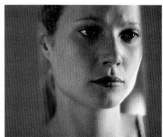

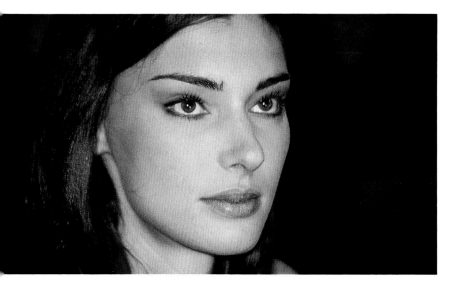

IDENTIFYING YOUR IMMUTABLE BEAUTY TRAIT:
IMPERFECT PERFECTION

Personal beauty style can be expressed in one striking feature—flawless skin, amazing hair, breathtaking eyes. Or it can be communicated through one's personality, ready smile, or great physical energy. In some cases, beauty style is defined by one's special aura, grace, or athleticism. To express your own beauty style, think about the following three steps:

1. Put yourself in an objective state of mind and identify that which is special about you. Ask your best friend, sister, or husband to help you identify your own unique beauty. Realize what is special about your looks. This could be almost anything—a few such characteristics are listed below.
2. Accept the features that you have and learn to feel good about them.
3. Start to play them up.

The idea is to accentuate the positive—whatever it is about you that is positive. There is a quality about each of us that makes us powerful and strong. For a woman with plain features, beauty style might come through in her mass of auburn hair. I know girls or women who look quite ordinary, yet I start to see them as beautiful because of their strength of character or elegance as a person. Likewise, there are models who, by acting in a rude or unpleasant way, stop looking pretty to my eye.

For some women, it's the ability to put on a red lipstick and wear it boldly. Being perceived as pretty is ultimately about exuding self-confidence. Self-confidence is the most elemental and yet most elusive quotient of beauty. I recognize instantly whether a woman possesses it—how at ease, how comfortable she is in her own skin. Oftentimes, the women with the most self-confidence seem to have other priorities in life and do not obsess endlessly about their looks.

I know from experience behind my makeup counter at Bergdorf Goodman—a shop on 57th Street in Manhattan that's a hub of luxury—that self-confidence is never a given. There I observe women with the most beautiful clothes and all the money in the world—but it doesn't mean that they are happy with their looks. If you don't feel good with yourself, nothing else matters. Maybe that's the key for all of us. Below I have listed specific striking beauty traits and more general beauty "looks" around which a woman can develop her own beauty style. You may find yourself identifying with one or perhaps even several of these categories—no matter. The point is that you are not alone. It can be tremendously reassuring and refreshing to see how many of the world's "greatest beauties" have the very same features the rest of us agonize over!

Round Face: It is a mistake to try to sculpt in cheekbones with makeup. Instead, line your eyes or play with lip colors and rejoice in the knowledge that you will always have a young appearance thanks to your face shape. Models often have this trait, which is one of the reasons they photograph so well.

Inspirations: Joan Chen, Andie MacDowell, Isabella Rossellini

Strong Nose: I find distinctive noses to be a regal and powerful element of beauty. It is one trait, however, that you may not like about yourself as a teenager but will surely grow into and love as an adult. Do not try to shade the nose or change it with makeup—that will only make your nose look like it is smudged with dirt.

Inspirations: Diana Vreeland, Anjelica Huston, Barbra Streisand

"Bedroom" Hooded Eyes: Women complain about hooded eyes all the time. I find them to be sexy and mysterious. Do not use dark shadow on the lid in an attempt to make your eyes stand out more—that will only blacken and further recess them. Instead, line your eyes with a stroke wide enough to still be visible when your eyes are open. A slight contour to eyes with light/medium shadow is a good technique to try. And don't forget to use a well-shaped brow to achieve good overall eye definition.

Inspirations: Charlotte Rampling, Tatjana Patitz, Jacqueline Bisset

Big Lips: A most desirable, luscious trait that smaller-lipped women spend thousands of dollars trying to achieve via silicone injections. To emphasize this feature, play up your lips by wearing richly pigmented lip colors. The fact is, you can wear any lip color in the world and it will look great! Conversely, if you want to scale down the appearance of your mouth, use paler lip colors and skip lip pencil. You might do just a gloss or lip stain and play up your eyes.

Inspirations: Brigitte Bardot, Kim Basinger, Naomi Campbell, Christy Turlington (as well as most models)

Small Lips: Do not attempt to create a bigger mouth by pencil lining beyond the edge of your mouth—it tends to look silly. Instead, use a lip pencil to define your mouth, going to the full extent of your natural lip line. Wear light-to-medium colors on your mouth and put the focus on your eyes.

Inspirations: Liza Minnelli, Courteney Cox

Big-Statement Hair: Standout hair color, such as auburn, jet black, or white blond, can be an identifying beauty trait in and of itself. There is no reason not to heighten hair color with highlights or a natural color rinse.

The key to making peace with your hair is to stop fighting its natural texture. If you have beautiful gray hair, accentuate it with a simple, sleek cut. Let the texture be as it is—perms tend to look old-fashioned. If you have the curliest hair in the world, just go with it. Find the best products around to manage any frizz but don't attempt to straighten hair. If your hair is straight naturally, accentuate its straightness by blowing it out smooth and working in high-shine styling products.

The true test of a great haircut is the ability to wash your hair, comb it, and go out without lengthy styling measures. The best haircut is one that suits the texture of your hair so that you are not a slave to your blow dryer, curling iron, or hot rollers.

Inspirations: Ava Gardner, Rita Hayworth, and Lucille Ball, for accentuating their redness; Marilyn Monroe and Madonna, for their unrelentingly platinum hair; Christie Brinkley, for her overwhelming blondness; Goldie Hawn, for her trademark golden hair; Farrah Fawcett, for her feminine, fluffy curls; Andie MacDowell, for making tight curls modern; and Linda Evangelista, for breaking hair-color convention by going whatever color(s) she chooses, whenever the mood hits.

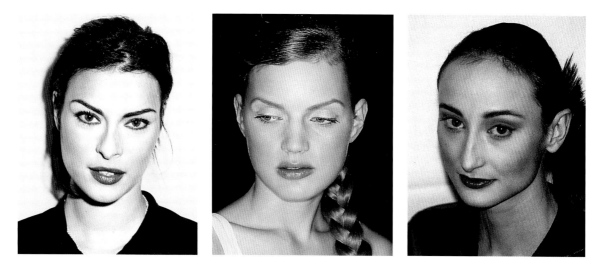

Big-Statement Eyes: Make your eyes your big statement and tone down your mouth with paler colors. Emphasize blue eyes with brown liner for day or navy liner for night. Don't wear blue eye shadow. Dark, exotic eyes should be made to smolder, with brown shadow (experiment with a wide range of browns) and charcoal or mahogany liner. Green eyes look even greener with khaki, pale yellow, or yellow-toned brown eye shadows. Use red-brown or charcoal liner and black mascara. In general, a charcoal, smudged liner makes any eye look more powerful.

Inspirations: blue eyes—Meg Ryan; brown eyes—Judy Garland, Ali MacGraw; green eyes—Vivien Leigh; violet eyes—Elizabeth Taylor.

Pale Skin: So many women with pale skin search for the perfect bronzing powder; instead, just make yourself as pale and soft as you can. Never go into the sun.

Inspirations: Bernadette Peters, Winona Ryder, Gwyneth Paltrow, Nicole Kidman, Shalom Harlow, Guinevere

Irregular Teeth: It is never too late to get braces, even if you are an adult. Clear braces are an option, and it's likely to be only a one-year commitment. A gap between your top front teeth, however, can be really appealing. You may want to choose not to get it fixed.

Inspiration: Lauren Hutton

Freckles: Visible freckles send the message of youth and freshness. I love to see freckles, and when I do the makeup for someone who is freckled, I much prefer letting them show through. Besides, women with freckles frequently have such extraordinary skin that they do not need the coverage of foundation. Instead of wearing orange lips and blush that "match" your complexion, try going in the opposite direction with pink tones.

If you choose to wear foundation, select one that is one shade darker than your skin tone (i.e., the same color as your freckles).

Inspirations: Picabo Street, Sissy Spacek, Patti Hansen, Bridget Hall

Moles/Birthmarks: Early in her career, Cindy Crawford was probably advised to have her mole removed. I myself had a mole removed when I was twenty after years of hating it. Cindy didn't listen and her mole has become a signature feature.

Inspirations: Marilyn Monroe, Cindy Crawford

Deep-Set Eyes: Lining eyes with a fine, dark line is the best way to open deep-set eyes. Avoid dark colors on the lid—use light to medium shadows instead. Apply highlighter at brow bone.

Inspirations: Jodie Foster, Demi Moore, Helen Hunt (and me!)

Big Brows: Don't be tempted to change your brow shape since a weighty eyebrow probably complements your features and frame. Instead, work on better defining your eyebrows. Pluck away any hairs between the brows and brush brow hairs up (using a firm toothbrush). If brows are sparse in spots, fill in using shadow and brow brush. (See chapter 12.)

Inspirations: Jacqueline Onassis, Brooke Shields, Ali MacGraw, Mariel Hemingway

Handsome Good Looks: Strong, handsome features can themselves constitute a signature beauty style. Opt for bold red or plum tones over dainty pink lip and blush colors. Dress in a simple style, avoiding excessively feminine frills and prints.

Inspirations: Katharine Hepburn, Emma Thompson, Coco Chanel, the Duchess of Windsor, Diana Vreeland, Lauren Bacall, K. D. Lang

Fresh, Natural Beauty: Wholesome good looks can be a defining beauty style. Focus on warm, golden tones to complement your look. Fresh natural beauty is often as much about a quick smile or good personality as anything.
Inspirations: Meg Ryan, Kelly Klein, Ali MacGraw, Candice Bergen

Classic Beauty: Simple but breathtaking. Beauty style should be effortless and minimal.

Inspirations: Grace Kelly, Sharon Stone, Julia Ormond, Slim Keith, Catherine Deneuve

Dark, Exotic Beauty: The sexiest kind of beauty. To emphasize, keep everything smoldering. Stick to dark colors—pastels and pale colors do not work. Be sure to match foundation to skin tone—do not go lighter.

Inspirations: Talisa Soto, Gloria Estefan, Yasmeen Ghauri, Sophia Loren

Athleticism: If you are strong and fit, this might be the basis of your beauty style. Chances are you look best in minimal—or even no—makeup. You can wear sleeveless dresses even in the middle of winter, because your athleticism will carry you through.

Inspirations: Gabrielle Reece, Mariel Hemingway, Gabriela Sabatini, Jackie Joyner-Kersee

Delicate Features: Play up your fine features with soft makeup (pastel tones, apricots, and baby pinks all work well). Eyebrows should be equally fine. Don't use harsh or high-contrast to define eye, brow, or mouth.

Inspirations: Babe Paley, Mia Farrow, Kate Moss, Michelle Pfeiffer, Audrey Hepburn, Twiggy

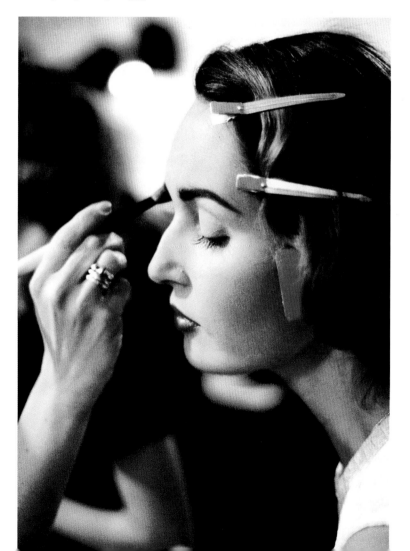

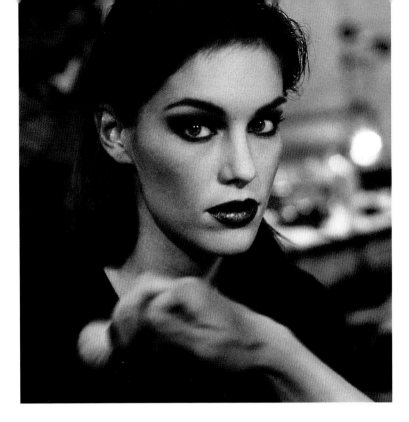

Extreme Height: As preteens and teenagers, most tall young women hate looking gawky and standing a head taller than the boys in their class. Later in life, however, a tall stature is an amazing asset. Maintain good posture to show off your height.

Inspirations: Sigourney Weaver, Uma Thurman, Princess Diana

Large Size: If you are overweight, makeup can play an important role in maintaining or building self-confidence. As anyone who has gained weight has probably experienced, your first reaction might be to do absolutely nothing for yourself, which, in the end, just makes you look and feel worse. Instead you should take the time to pull yourself together, wear makeup, and get your hair done. If you start feeling good from the top, soon you will start feeling good all the way down.

It is important to accept that people come in all different sizes—thin, medium, and big. Each of us must accept the frame we were born with: Some people are simply big-boned. Instead of looking at skinny models for fashion and beauty inspiration, try to find someone with your same shape. Some women are born to be big, and should feel beautiful for that.

Inspirations: large-size models

COSMETIC SURGERY

I truly believe that you can change how you feel about your features—even those things you might now hate. In general, it's a much better thing to accept the looks you have. If there is something that makes you feel truly horrible, such as facial moles, and if there is a safe and uncomplicated way to change it, then that may prove to be the best course of action. I have a friend who so hated her droopy eyes that she had them surgically lifted. At the time, I wished she had not done it. When I saw how much happier she was for it, I accepted that it was the right thing for her.

A decision like this should never be rash. (Lots of women who got radical nose jobs in the 1970s regretted it later.) Do your homework to find the best doctors. Then give yourself plenty of time to think it over.

HERE AND NOW BEAUTY

"God, I looked so great!" I hear this all the time. Women bring along a favorite picture of themselves—dog-eared from wear—and ask me how they can regain that look. Usually, the picture was taken years ago. My response tends to be: "Well, of course you looked great! You were eighteen years old."

Focus on the here and now. It doesn't matter if you looked gorgeous ten years ago when you were in your teens or twenties. Dwelling on the past is not really healthy or useful. It is important to appreciate where you are now. You are at a different place in your life now—celebrate that.

One of the easiest ways of looking younger and more modern is simply by doing less: Wear less jewelry, and choose clothing that has simpler lines and fewer patterns. Wear makeup to look healthy, not artificial.

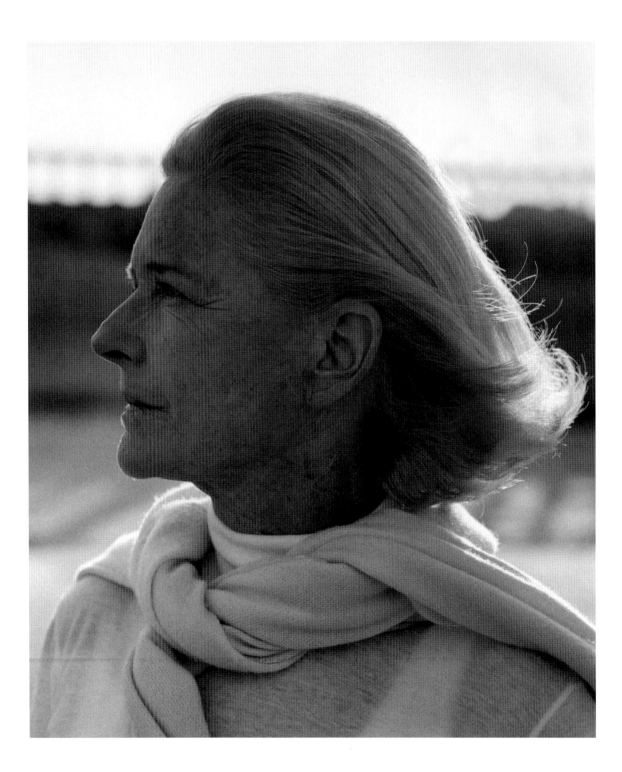

6

WOMEN WITH EXTRAORDINARY BEAUTY STYLE

I have encountered countless women with natural beauty style. Even seen from afar, real beauty style speaks to me instantly and always intrigues me. I have chosen a small number of these women to illustrate the concept of developing and possessing your own beauty style. Beyond simply looking flawless or great, the members of this group of women have long inspired me with their individualism and confidence. In each case, I believe that there is an inner beauty just as bright as their outer, physical beauty traits. That, in the end, is how I define real beauty.

C. Z. Guest (left) is a regal beauty whose style centers on an elegant simplicity. For her, the most basic minimal makeup is as appropriate for an afternoon in her garden as it is for a tony society gala. That fact alone reveals the strength of her beauty style.

Tina Turner (right) possesses a peaceful, spiritual kind of beauty. Her features themselves are strong, but her soul is kind and soft. The tension between her inner and outer beauty is fascinating to me. Most of us are familiar with Tina made up in a strong, stagy kind of way. But for this picture, I underdid the makeup so that the inner Tina would shine through.

Lucie de la Falaise (below) has a sweet sort of beauty. I love her best when she smiles, because her dimples are adorable and her face lights up so beautifully. There's something offbeat about her looks: She manages to look uptown and downtown at the same time.

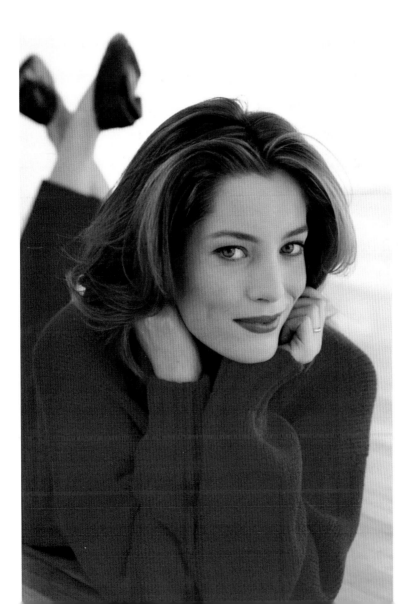

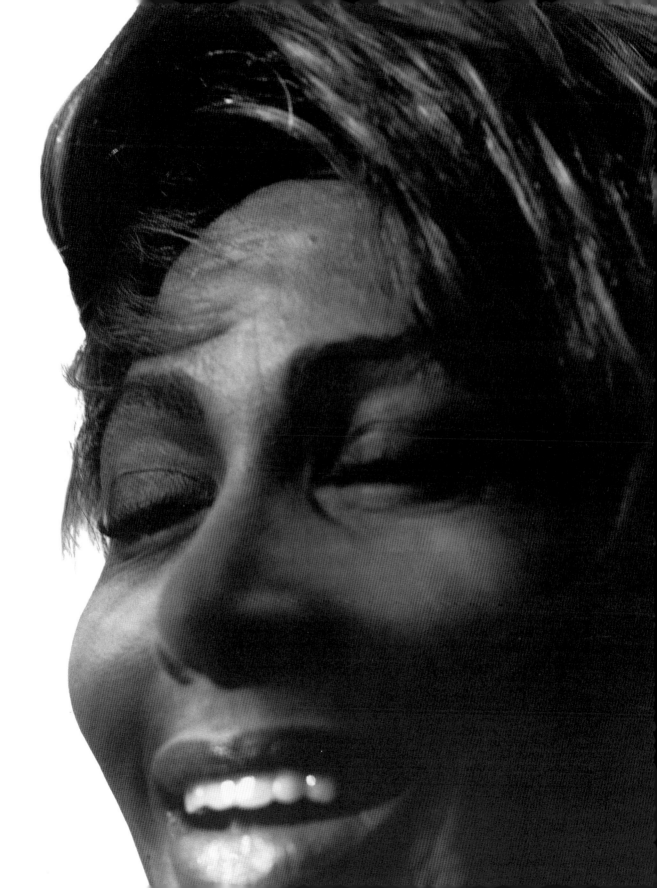

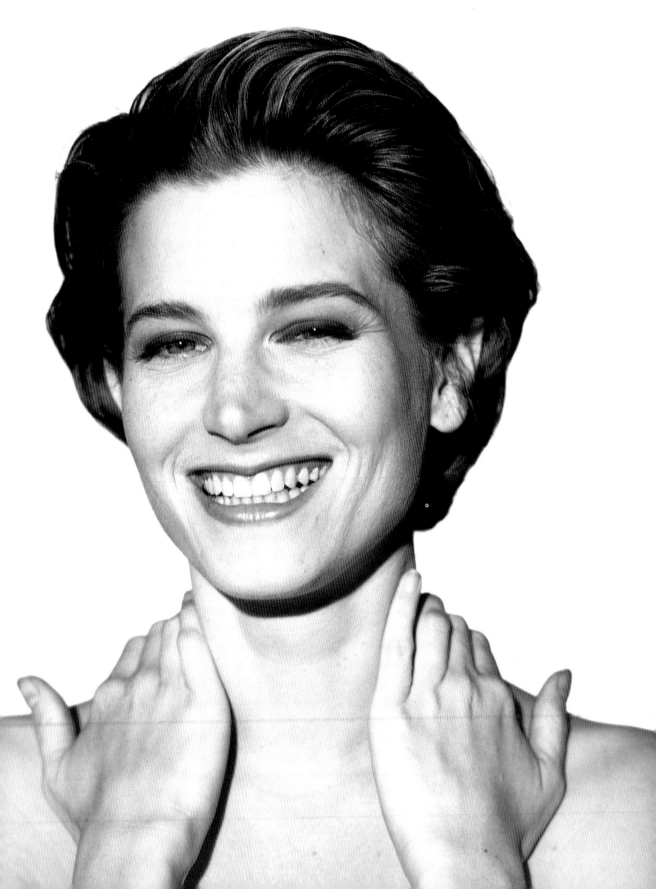

Bridget Fonda (far left) possesses a very delicate, sweet kind of beauty. That's not to say that she doesn't have a strong personality. I like to define Bridget's features without overpowering her softness and simplicity. I just try to keep it simple and let her pretty skin come through.

Anne Kampmann (below left) has a wonderful sense of humor and an amazingly fit body. Her beauty style stems from these two things, which is to say she looks best in the least amount of makeup. For Anne, day makeup means lip balm and evening makeup means tinted lip balm. It's that simple!

Lillian Wang (below) is a tawny, exotic beauty. Her skin is smooth perfection. Her style is simple and classic, but always current. I like to use deep, warm tones on her face to bring out the warm tones in her skin.

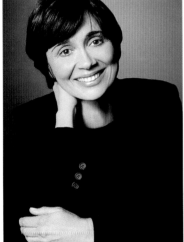

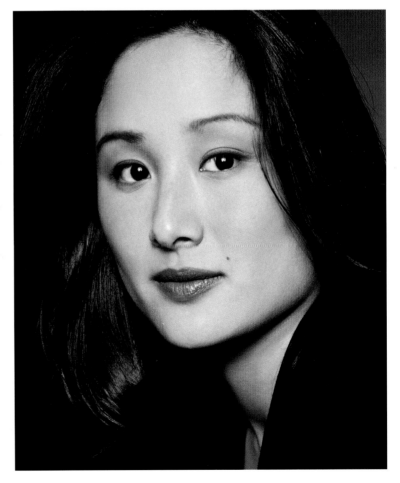

Linda Wells possesses an intelligent kind of beauty. She always looks perfectly simple and absolutely correct. Linda is an example of a porcelain beauty, where a little bit of makeup in pale colors is what looks best.

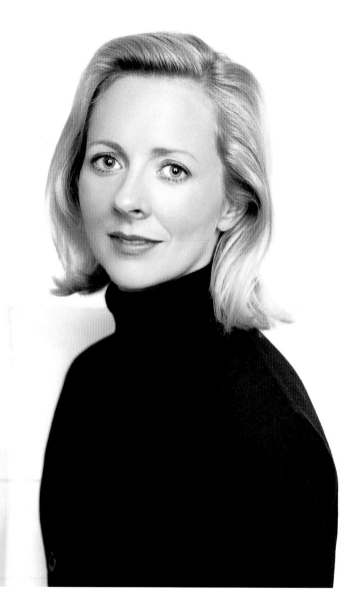

Joan Vass (below left) has a strong beauty that's defined by healthy, outdoorsy skin and her fabulous white hair. Her beauty style and personality are one.

Mary Randolph Carter (below right) is a cool beauty—she has piercing blue eyes, pale skin, and the softest pink cheeks—but has a casual style and a warm personality. The combination is powerful.

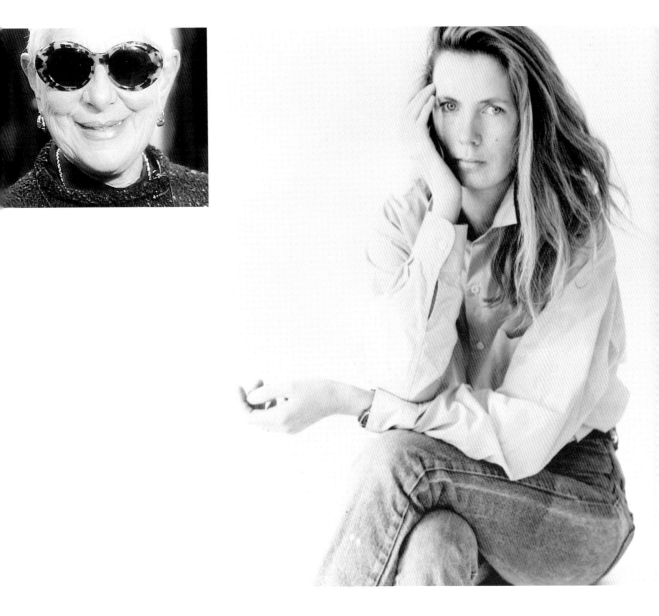

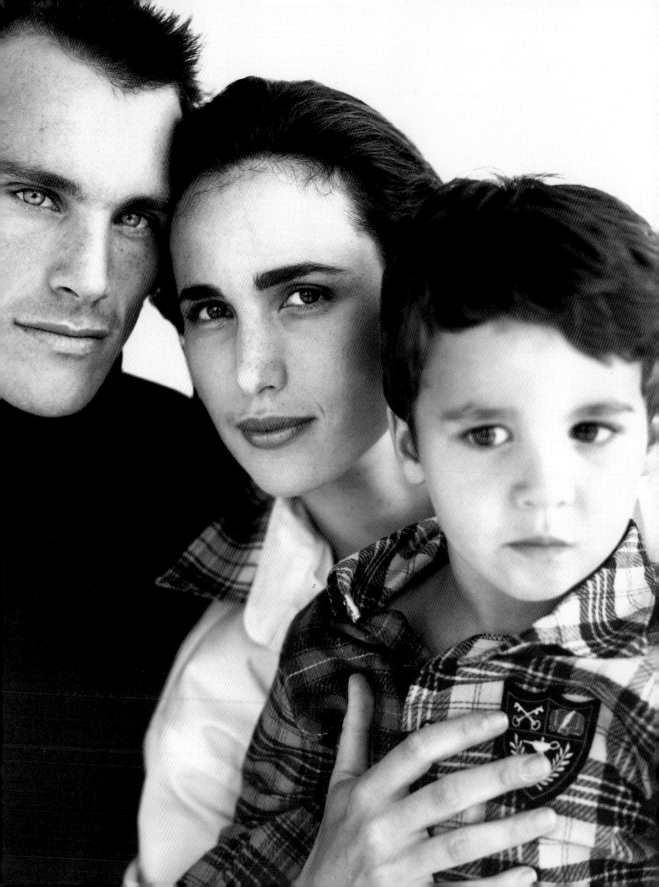

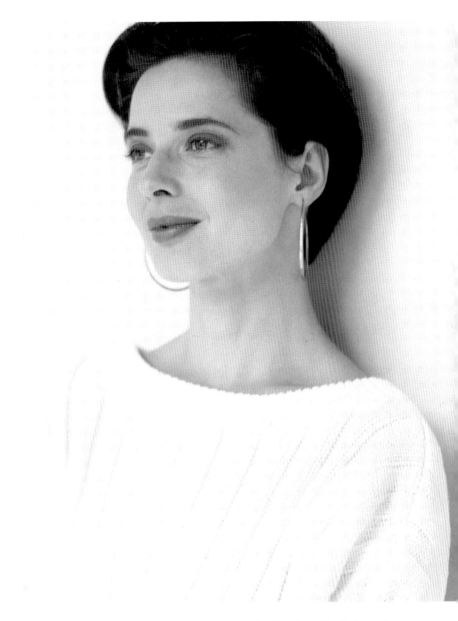

Isabella Rossellini (above) has the most breathtaking face. She is the quintessential chameleon: Makeup changes her entirely. But I love her best as is.

Andie MacDowell (left) is one of the great natural beauties of our time. Her lips, brows, and hair are lovely and distinctive. When you meet her, she intentionally puts you at ease with her sense of humor so that her incredible beauty is not overwhelming. (Here, Andie with her husband and son.)

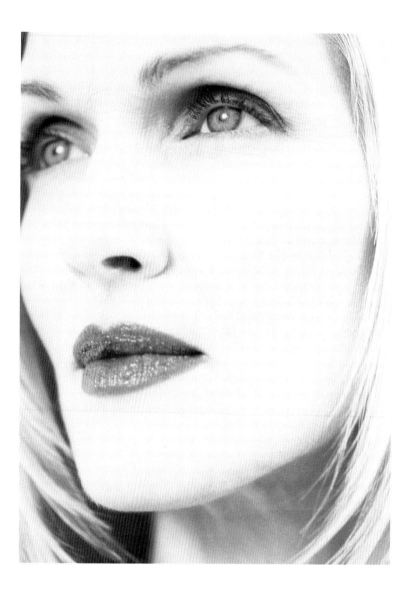

Dianne de Witt (above) has a refined, regal beauty that can be soft or very chiseled and powerful.

Ricky Lauren (right) is the epitome of outdoorsy, understated, timeless beauty. She has a clear idea of her own beauty style and never veers from that look. I love to do a bronzy, tan look on her—just heightening how she looks with no makeup. Put gloss on her lips and a bit of highlight for the evening, and she is truly elegant. She sparkles.

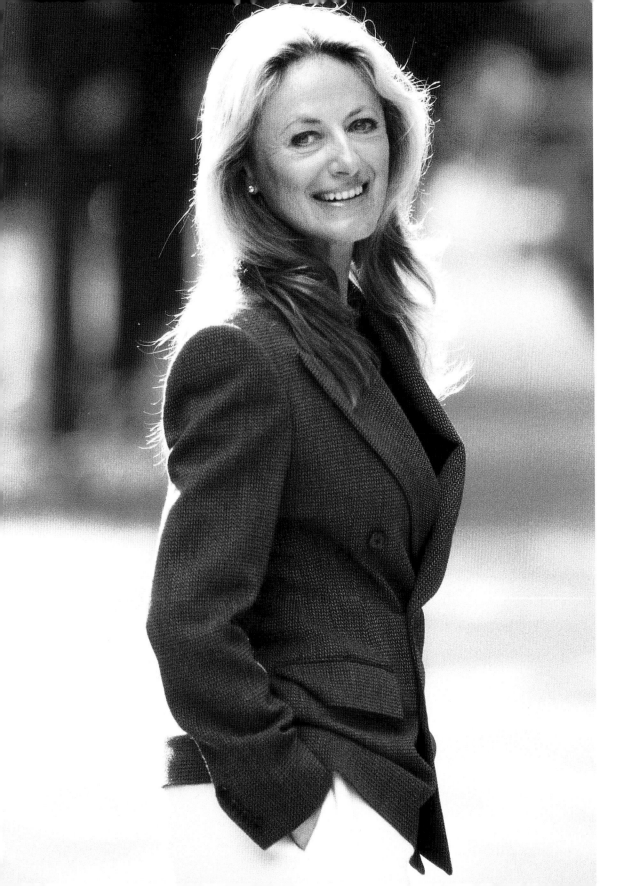

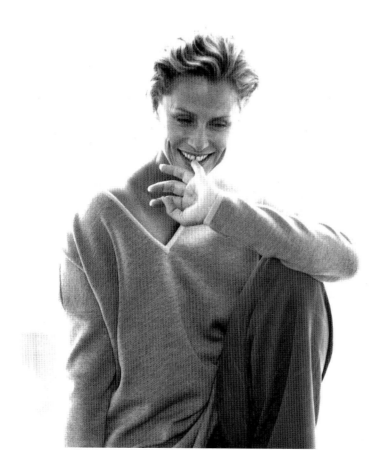

Lauren Hutton (above) has a self-assured beauty style. She always knows *who* she is, *where* she is going, and exactly *how* she wants to look.

Susan Sarandon (right) is a beauty chameleon—she likes to look glamorous and she likes to look natural. But given Susan's pared-down style, it is important that even glamorous makeup be kept simple; I like to do a red mouth or a smoky eye. For a natural face, I like to do nude lips and pink cheeks that complement her warm coloring.

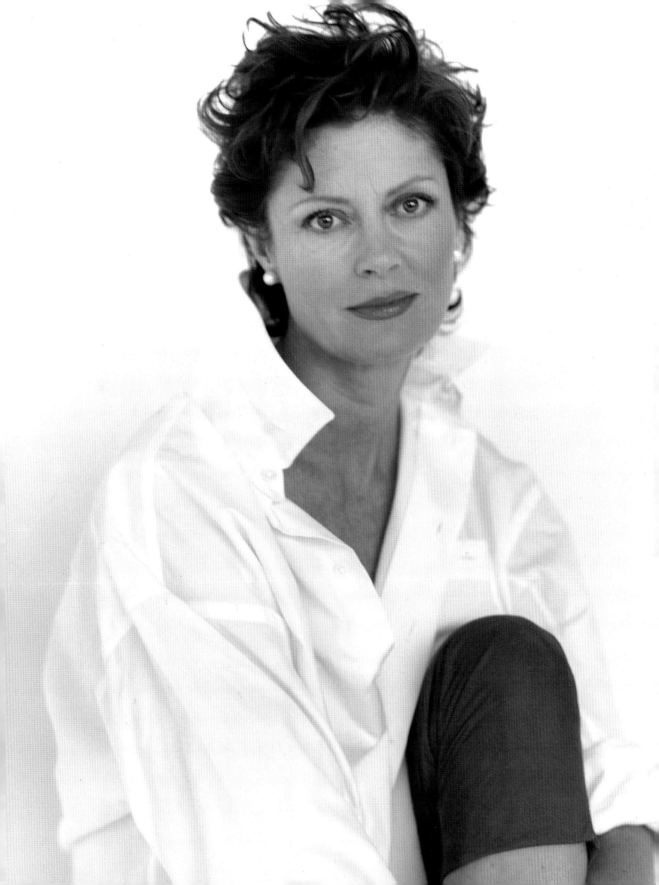

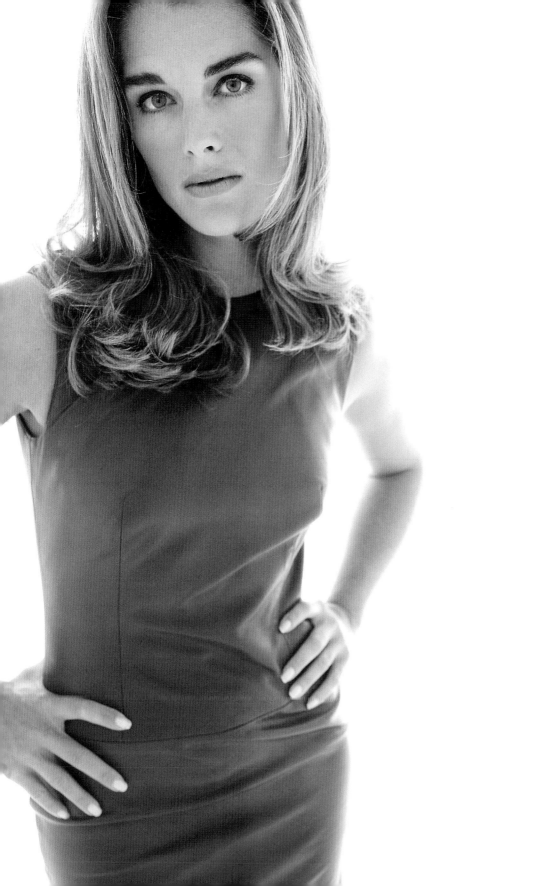

Brooke Shields (left) is as close to a perfect beauty as any I have ever encountered. Any makeup put on her face looks amazing. She is equally beautiful made up soft and clear or strong and trendy. And of course I love her gorgeous eyebrows, which triggered the rage for thick, unkempt brows in the late 1970s. Just think of the influence Brooke has had, considering that she is still a young woman!

Paloma Picasso (below) is a classic, strong beauty. Her look is unmistakable and perfectly unique. She defines the strength of a red-lipstick personality.

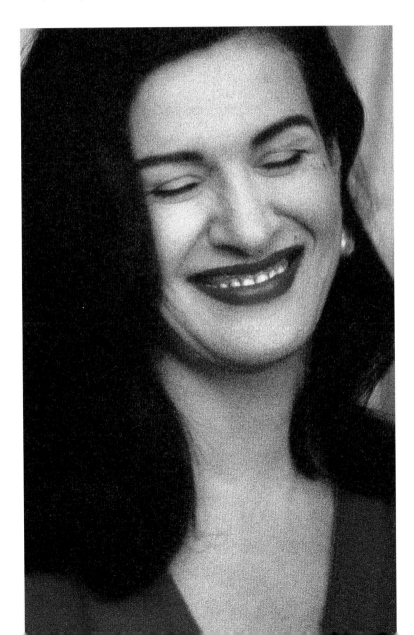

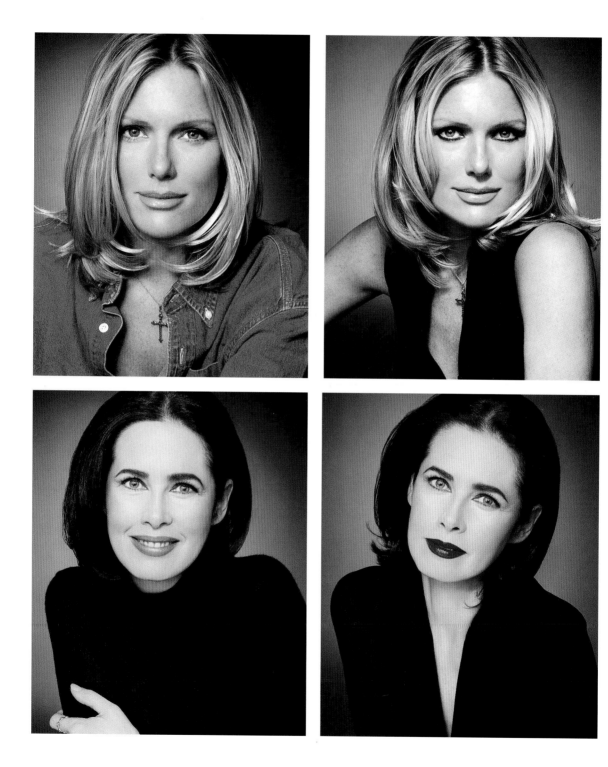

7

IN SEARCH OF YOUR OWN BEAUTY STYLE

I've always made a practice of looking at women. It's sort of a private mission to survey as many women as I can, whether I'm walking down the streets of New York City, waiting for a plane at O'Hare Airport in Chicago, or grocery shopping in suburban New Jersey. It's a great way to learn about beauty and fashion style. It is not an envious or jealous sort of observation—we've all had the uncomfortable experience of being obviously looked up and down by another woman out of insecurity or jealousy—instead, I look in a nonjudgmental, sometimes even admiring, way and ask myself: What does she do that I can learn from? How is it that she puts her hair in a ponytail so that it doesn't look sloppy or teenaged, but easy and sophisticated? Why do her stockings work so well with her shoes? Why does her shade of lipstick look so pretty? Why does she look good?

You can apply the same rules of observation to characters on television or in the movies. (This is much more useful than looking at supermodels for style direction.) The idea is to be realistic with whom you look at—choose someone who is close to your age and shape. If your body is a little rounder, don't look at someone who is string-bean thin for swimsuit ideas. Magazines that have stories about real people can be useful style-scanners.

Developing your own beauty style means prioritizing what matters most to you and what makes you feel good. For me, comfort is number one. Simplicity and practicality come next. Looking good comes in third, which is very clear to me on the days I am driving into the city trying to put on my makeup at stoplights.

If looking good is your number-one priority, you'll want to budget more time for your makeup—fifteen to twenty minutes. You should plan to do it in front of a serious mirror, with as much natural light as possible, and have at your fingertips all your tools, brushes, and makeup.

Even with priorities clearly in mind, many women become frustrated or overwhelmed with the world of beauty. They desire to look their best, but just don't know quite where to begin. This is a most basic issue for women; if you identify with these feelings, you are not alone. Here are four of the most common beauty-stagnant situations I have found—each with plans of action for moving forward with your looks.

Scenario One: The Makeup Virgin

- You are stunned that you have somehow reached adulthood without the first clue about wearing makeup.
- You want a more sophisticated, polished look but are not willing to make a big-time or makeup commitment.
- Your makeup skills are remedial to nil.
- You've always been uncomfortable with the idea of makeup and foundation.

Start slowly. It's unlikely that you will feel comfortable going from natural to a totally made-up look. A traditional department store makeover is not advisable, since it might involve too overwhelming and dramatic a transformation.

Instead, I suggest focusing on the two most basic elements: finding a foundation and powder that match your skin tone and a lip color or stain that matches your natural lip color perfectly. These are the two hardest, but ultimately most satisfying, elements of makeup.

Scenario Two: The Color Addict

- You wear bright makeup—colorful lipstick, bright blusher—and feel that you need a strong jolt of color.
- You would try more muted tones, but you are afraid of looking too plain and un-made-up.

It might be hard for your eye to adjust to a quieter palette of makeup, but ultimately you will see for yourself that more natural tones do look more sophisticated and modern. Natural makeup doesn't mean a drab or no-makeup look: Natural simply means using the correct tones for your skin.

The hardest thing is deciding where to start. It's always a good idea to examine your foundation. Is it too white or too pink? With a warmer, more yellow-toned foundation, skin looks more natural and even bright colors look their best. The next step would be to choose one element of makeup to tone down. If you wear a bright green eye shadow, for example, try a more muted shade like moss green. If you wear fuchsia lipstick, try mixing it with a brown-based pink.

If, on the other hand, bold makeup colors work for you and have become your defined element of beauty style, stick with them. If you love wearing bright, bright lipstick and it makes you feel really great, then that's your statement. Just be extra careful that your foundation and powder match your face perfectly, that they are not pink-toned, and that you use only as much as you really need.

There are some combinations that are extremely pretty: A woman with jetblack hair, for example, can look gorgeous wearing fuchsia lipstick. A woman with gray hair can look beautiful wearing bright orange on her lips.

Scenario Three: Stuck in a Rut

- You haven't changed anything about your look since high school.
- You, and everyone around you, is bored with your look.

Start with a serious new haircut. Make an appointment for a consultation with a top hairdresser in your community. (If you are unsure which salon to go to, ask a friend—or even a complete stranger whose hair you like.) The point of the consultation is to hear the hairstylist's recommendation and also to see whether you feel comfortable with this person. Remember that you are in control of this situation. Do not do the cut on the spot, even if you love the idea of the cut. Think it over, then schedule your appointment.

A modern, updated cut is usually about a quite simple shape. It is generally wise not to have lots of layers cut in, which tend to look either old-fashioned or too trendy. A measure of a haircut is that it looks good after it is washed and air-dried—without styling tools or blow-dryers. It's useful to have a nonstyling option for weekends and holidays.

Beautiful hair today is all about texture. Whether your hair is silky smooth, stick-straight, wavy, or full of corkscrew curls, the idea is to push your natural texture to its most beautiful. If your hair is straight, blow it out so that it looks shiny, smooth, and perfectly straight. If your hair is wavy, work gel into the waves as they dry. I am not a believer in permanent waves or body waves, because they can damage hair and alter its natural texture. I have ruined my hair more than once in this way, so I speak from experience! In fact, many top salons in Manhattan recommend against perms; some even refuse to do them.

Once you have a new hairstyle, it's time to go to a makeup expert. A good approach is to enter a department store and look for a sales associate behind the counter whose makeup you especially like. Then approach that person with specific questions in mind, such as how to better wear concealer, how to brighten your face with blush, etc. Some makeup counters will prescribe a full face of makeup—whatever you do, don't feel obliged to wear everything they advise. It is probably too much information to retain, anyhow. Ask for the most simple beginner's approach or for what you most want to know, then return if you want to add on.

Scenario Four: You Want to Feel Pretty Again

- You feel drab and unattractive.
- You have just experienced an illness or an emotional trauma and you feel that your looks have changed irrevocably.
- You see little that you like when you look in the mirror.
- You find yourself focusing on all that is negative.

If you find yourself obsessing over wrinkles in the mirror, perhaps your bathroom lighting is too cruel. Work to create lighting that is more flattering to you. Try a lower-wattage bulb for starters. Airplane bathrooms have notoriously unflattering mirrors. Every pore and wrinkle stands out so loud and clear that you cannot help but fixate on your imperfections. Remember, we all have imperfections, and we must simply accept them as part of who we are.

I use daylight as much as possible. My bathroom at home is designed to allow in as much natural light as possible. Mirrors are an important consideration, too. I once lived in an apartment where the mirror sat tilted on the floor at the most flattering angle (I was too busy to hang it properly). Every day just before going out, I would look at myself in the mirror and get a boost. It made me look tall and thin, and even though I knew the "lie of the mirror," it always put me in a good mood.

If you have just suffered an illness or an emotional upset, it's a good idea to take some time for yourself. Go on a trip to visit an old friend or a favorite relative. Go alone or with a best friend to a spa for a week, or commit to a new exercise program that will boost your energy. Most important, do not feel selfish for lavishing attention on yourself. You need and deserve it now more than ever.

There are other times, however, when the only thing that works is to put your beauty on hold. Just ignore it. You need this time to reflect and do anything but dwell on your looks. In times of trouble, beauty shouldn't be your number-one priority. When you are ready, you can go back to it.

YOUR MAKEUP PERSONALITY: TWO SURVEYS

ARE YOU IN A MAKEUP RUT?

1. Do you attempt to re-create the makeup look you had in a favorite old photograph of yourself? If so, when was the picture taken?

2. Have you ever tried to purchase a favorite lipstick or eye shadow only to find that the shade has been discontinued?

3. Do you follow the same basic makeup routine every day regardless of the occasion, the season, or the clothes you're wearing?

4. Do you feel naked without mascara?

5. Do you feel naked without eyeliner?

6. Have you had the same exact hairstyle for at least the past five years?

7. Do you always wear makeup? About how many waking hours per week do you spend not wearing makeup?

8. Do you use dark brown lip pencil to line your mouth?

9. Do you wear the same makeup you wore in high school? Have you worn the same makeup for the past five years?

10. Have you always worn frost?

11. Have you noticed that a favorite lip or eye color has made a comeback?

12. Do you buy the same lipstick shade again and again?

13. Have you always worn three eye shadow shades at a time?

14. Do you wear red lipstick all the time—to the gym, with a swimsuit, everywhere?

Score

Question one: If you try to re-create the look, take 1 point. If the picture was taken in the last year, take 0 points. If the picture is older than that, take 1 point for each year the picture is old. (If you don't have a favorite picture of yourself, take 0 points.)

Questions 2–6: Take one point for each yes answer.

Question 7: Take one point if your answer is yes. If you spend less than 10 waking hours/week not wearing makeup, take one extra point.

Questions 8–13: Take one point for each yes response.

Question 14: If you answered yes, you are a red lipstick personality. I consider red lipstick to be a category of makeup unto itself. It is completely timeless and always in fashion. If you wear red lipstick religiously, you are automatically not in a rut—you have found your own true beauty style.

Analysis

If you scored:

0–3: You are definitely not stuck in a makeup rut. Proceed to beauty addict quiz, which follows.

4–5: Your makeup routine is stagnant. Consult how-to chapters to gather some new ideas and learn to be more creative.

6 or more: Your makeup is living in the past. It's probably a good idea to start all over. Start with a makeup cleanup (see chapter 8).

ARE YOU A BEAUTY ADDICT?

1. Do you buy makeup on a monthly basis?

2. Is there some item of makeup in every room of your home?

3. Do you reread makeup stories in magazines?

4. Do you spend more time reading *Allure* magazine than you do reading the newspaper?

5. Do you always buy the latest hot beauty product?

6. Do you know the names of three (or more) celebrity makeup artists?

7. Do you know the shade names of your lipsticks?

8. Do two or more cosmetics salespeople at your favorite department store know you by name?

9. Are you never completely happy with the way you look?

10. Are you impatient for next season's colors to arrive at the makeup counter?

Analysis

If you answered yes to more than four of the above questions, you qualify as a beauty addict.

The first thing to do—painful as it may seem—is force yourself to come clean on how much money you spend on makeup. Check your store bills and credit-card receipts for the past few months. If you find you are buying makeup weekly or monthly, it's really a problem—and completely unnecessary. A dependence on makeup may be masking a feeling of inadequacy. Occasionally buying makeup on impulse is a perfectly natural and fun outlet. But if your automatic response to an ugly day or to a sad or difficult situation is to buy beauty products, then plan a strategy for the next time you experience a purchasing pang. Go to the gym instead. Get a massage. Or meet a friend for coffee. It may end up costing you the same amount of money, but it will be better for your well-being.

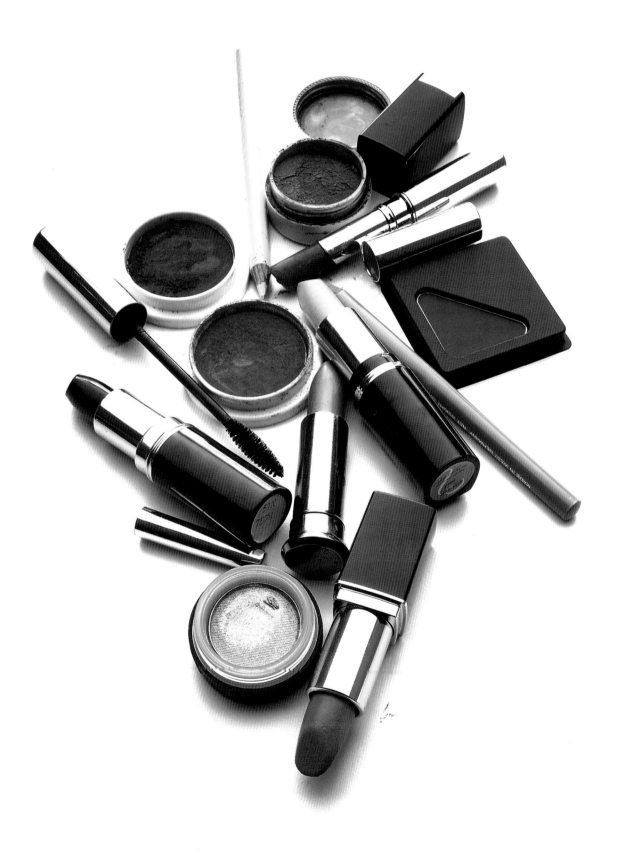

8

MAKEUP ORGANIZATION

Full-Disclosure Makeup Analysis

This may sound like a painful exercise, but it's guaranteed to simplify your makeup wardrobe faster than anything. It will also keep you from spending money on things you already own or repeating the common mistake of buying products that you never use.

Gather up all the makeup products in your life—your essentials from the bathroom cabinet or vanity table, your ancillary items stuck in various tote bags and pocketbooks, coat and jacket pockets, and from the glove compartment. Dump everything on the floor and arrange like products together, i.e., put all lipsticks in one pile; foundations in another; shadows in another; pencil liners in another; and so on.

- Toss anything that you've had for two years or longer (see "Expiration Dates").
- Smell everything. Toss anything that has a funny or musty odor.
- Toss anything that's chipped, messy, or runny.
- Throw out brushes that are falling apart and puffs and sponges that are dirty or falling apart.
- Check to see if any liquids have separated. If so, dispose of them.
- Throw out anything that you have not touched in the past six months—even that perfect red lipstick you've been saving. If you haven't found an occasion to wear it now, you probably won't ever—like the aqua eye shadow you bought to match that aqua bridesmaid's dress. (I try to apply this same cleaning-out standard to my wardrobe.)
- Edit out any colors that are just plain ugly or garish.
- Throw out any colors that are pasty or dull-looking—shades that don't do anything for your skin tone.
- Weed out makeup that has a strong shimmer or frost.

Analyze what's left: What are the dominant colors? What are the products you use every day? What were the most obvious mistake purchases? The optimum makeup organization is to have two kits—your home supplies, from which you never steal for travel or daytime touch-ups, and your day kit/travel kit, which ideally comprises a stand-alone system in smaller sizes.

Expiration Dates

One of the most objective (and least agonizing!) ways of clearing excess products out of your life is to toss anything that's been open to the air too long to still be safe, clean, or effective. Below are some rule-of-thumb life spans for products once they've been opened.

- Cream cleanser   1 year
- Cream/moisturizer   1 year
- Foundation, oil-based   1.5 years
- Foundation, water-based   1 year
- Gel cleanser   1 year
- Lipstick   1–2 years
- Mascara   3–4 months
- Powder   2 years
- Shadows   2 years
- Brushes   wash every 2–3 months
- Sponges: wash weekly and discard monthly

Makeup Quarters

To avoid meltdown, do not store products on a windowsill that gets light or in a steamy bathroom. Avoid leaving makeup in a parked car, which can get hot.

Resealable bags: I find that see-through plastic bags are the best possible makeup containers. They allow you to see everything that is inside, so you don't waste time rummaging around. They also force you to keep your makeup clean and neat, as everything is exposed. Best of all, they are inexpensive, disposable, and easy to replace. I organize my professional makeup kits using resealable bags, which are also great for travel. I couldn't live without them.

Slightly thicker plastic bags work nicely, too (drawstring bags, like marble bags, or flatter storage bags are available inexpensively at most drugstores). I like that they force organization. Buy two or three: one for skin products (concealer, concealer brush, foundation, powder, sponge, and powder puff); one for color (blush, eye shadows, eyeliners, lip pencils, mascara, and lip colors); and a third for tools (all brushes).

I really believe in makeup cleanliness—it helps me stay clearheaded and organized. I am fanatical about keeping my makeup clean and neat and about discarding things when they get messy, especially sponges and applicators. This way, it is so much easier to apply makeup and get out the door—everything is at your fingertips.

At home, I keep my makeup essentials on a table in the bathroom; extras go into drawers. I use metal cups to store pencils and brushes, and a Plexiglas organizer for lipsticks. Everything else is laid out on a tray. Some women like to keep makeup in a tackle box or toolbox, which is great since you can see everything when it's open; even better, you can put it away when it's closed. Other women line drawers with dividers so that makeup doesn't get jumbled. Find a system that works for you, but avoid the "dump" system, i.e., dumping all your products into a box—you'll be forever searching for something.

Makeup Day Kit

I like to have a separate set of essentials packed to carry with me all the time. This is especially useful on days when you can't make it home before going out at night.

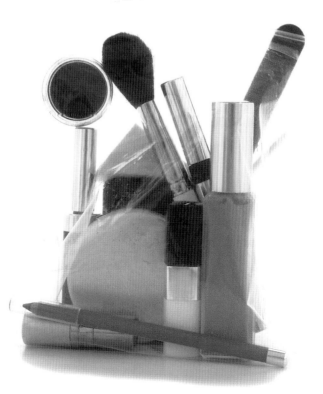

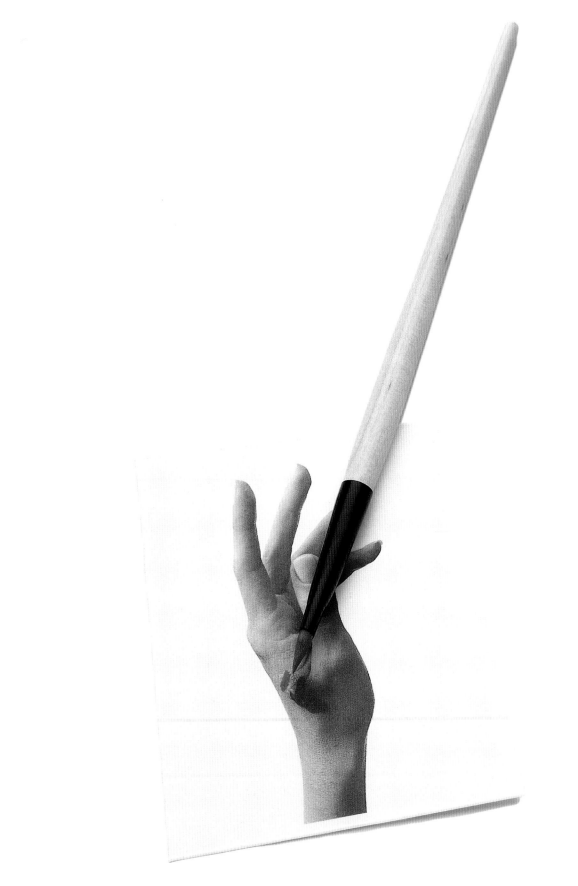

9

TOOLS

The right makeup tools are as important in getting the look you want as the actual makeup itself. The applicators included with most makeup are simply not up to the job. Blush brushes are usually too small and too coarse to enable you to place the color where you want it on the cheek and to blend it well enough to look natural. Bad blush brushes are the reason so many women go around wearing unattractive stripes of blush across their faces. Similarly, the sponge applicators that come with many eye shadow kits are difficult to hold and, for me, impossible to control. Nonetheless, tools are probably the most overlooked and underrated aspect of the process for most women.

Many women balk at the idea of buying separate tools—perhaps they feel that it's an extravagance or an unnecessary expense. I cannot emphasize enough the value of good makeup tools. Proper tools can make applying makeup much easier and faster. You will have greater control of your makeup and will be able to achieve a more natural and long-lasting look. I guarantee that good tools will make you much happier with the entire process. And remember, when properly cared for, good brushes can last years.

If the idea of makeup brushes is daunting to you, try buying only the four absolute essentials: concealer brush, shadow brush, eyeliner brush, and blush brush. (If you tend to wear bright or dark lip colors, you should also have a lip brush.) Then, using masking tape and a permanent marker, identify each of them. That way you will not get confused or frustrated in the mad rush to get yourself together in the morning.

How to know if a brush is good quality? Brushes should be soft and full and should feel comfortable in your hand. Run your hand through the bristles. It's a bad sign if they come out readily.

Makeup brushes are sold wherever makeup is sold—department stores, drugstores, and cosmetic-supply stores. Makeup artists' makeup lines often have good brushes. Brushes sold at art-supply stores are usually of the highest quality and are often sold at reasonable prices.

VELOUR POWDER PUFF

To press on face powder and "lock" foundation in place. Look for one that is roughly the size of your hand. It should be washed by hand weekly or biweekly and should last for six months, or more. A good puff is worth the investment since it will create a smoother finish to the face; it would also be washable so it should last up to six months. Good quality puffs are available at better drug or department stores.

SPONGE

Wedge-shaped, to smooth or blend in foundation. Buy a bag of latex ones (available inexpensively at most drugstores) and use each for about a week, then throw out. Larger, denser sponges (found at department stores)are also excellent and washable. Natural sea sponges are not a good option, since they tend to absorb too much foundation.

SHADOW BRUSH

A short brush, cut full and square for a clean sweep of color.

LINER BRUSH

A small, flat brush which is gently rounded to a point.

BLUSH BRUSH

A medium-full, round brush. It is tapered at the sides to allow for more controlled blending and usually has a long handle.

BROW BRUSH

Bristles are quite firm and are clipped at an angle to allow for clean, even application of shadow to the brows' coarse hairs.

TWEEZERS

I prefer metal ones that are angled at the end (as opposed to the pincer-point models). Note: This is a lifetime purchase, so don't scrimp here.

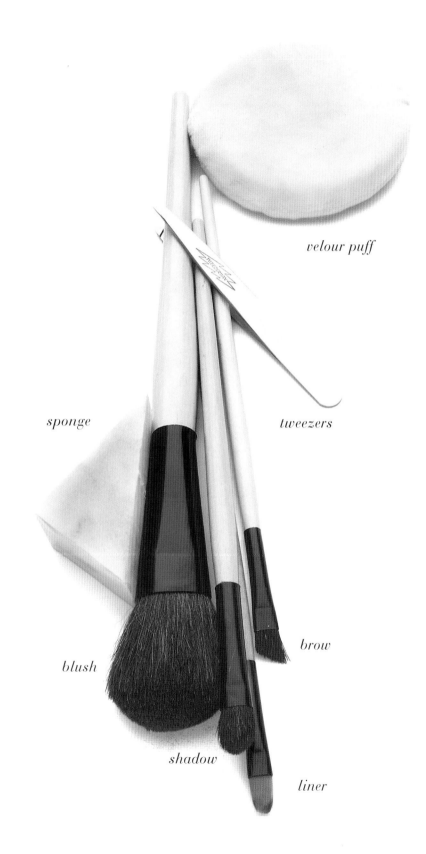

velour puff

sponge

tweezers

blush

shadow

brow

liner

À LA CARTE TOOLS

The nonessentials that you may want to try once a month, or once a year.

POWDER BRUSH

A big, fluffy brush to be used with face powder.

CONCEALER BRUSH

A narrow, firm brush works best (synthetic bristles are preferable here). It should be tapered to a flat head.

LIP BRUSH

Similar to a concealer brush except smaller. It should be firm and small. Look for a retractable version or one with a cap for cleanliness and portability.

EYELASH CURLER

A scissorslike apparatus with rubber pads that closes on lashes and causes them to turn up. The most basic curlers are the best option.

CONTOUR EYE BRUSH

Slightly wider, fatter, and firmer than the shadow brush. Its tapered edges allow center bristles to position shadow at corner of eye.

There are two other à la carte brushes (not pictured) that I quite like. Admittedly, they are specialty items. But if they sound useful to you, they are probably worth the investment.

BRONZING POWDER BRUSH

A fat, full brush to be used with a dark powder for an overall glow. It usually has a short, thick handle.

BLENDER BRUSH

Soft, loose, fluffy, and relatively large. Takes the edge off color.

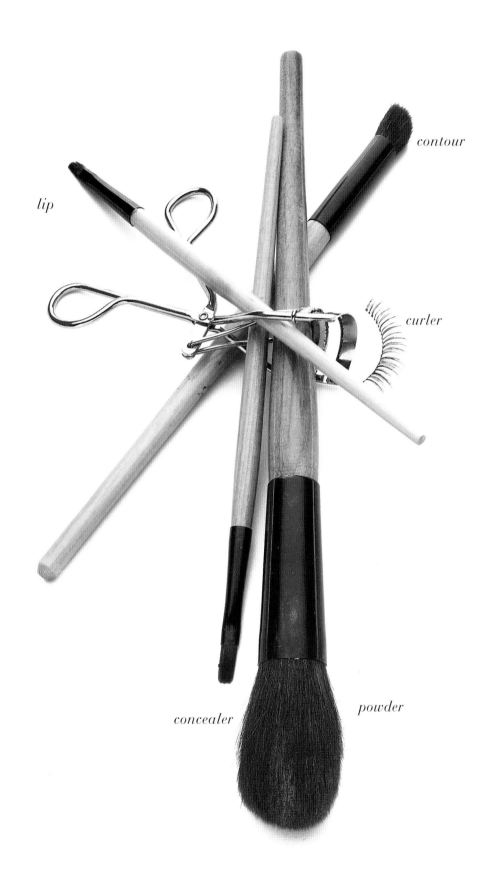

lip

contour

curler

concealer

powder

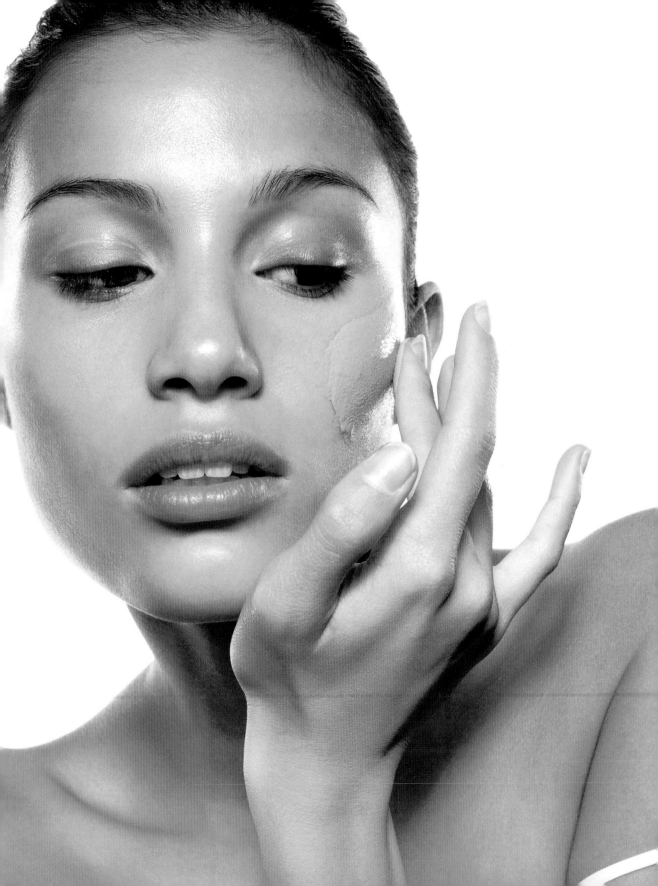

HOW TO WASH BRUSHES

To clean makeup brushes, use a mild household liquid soap (baby shampoo and Ivory soap work well). Use your hand as a cup for the warm, soapy water and swirl brushes in your palm until they are clean. Rinse well. Then gently squeeze excess water from the brush. Reshape the head of the brush. Air-dry by laying the brush over the edge of a counter or table so that the bristles are open to the air on all sides. Brushes should dry overnight.

There is absolutely no need to buy a special makeup-brush cleaning solution. Most solutions specifically made for this purpose are too harsh and drying for the bristles. I've found that some of these solutions have an odd odor. Rubbing alcohol is not a good option, either—it too is drying.

Do not soak brushes in the sink. Extended immersion in water can loosen the glue that holds the bristles in place, so brushes come apart prematurely. Also, to avoid mildew from forming, do not wrap your brushes in, or lay them on, a towel to dry.

TRICKS OF THE TRADE

Your Hands: A makeup artist's hands are his/her most precious tool. I use my hands to warm concealers, blend foundation, or mix two lip shades. I also use my hands to work makeup into my face, or my subject's face, so that the makeup feels like a part of the face and not like a mask. Your face should never feel "untouchable," even when it is fully made-up. The more comfortable you become using your hands on your face, the more natural your makeup will look.

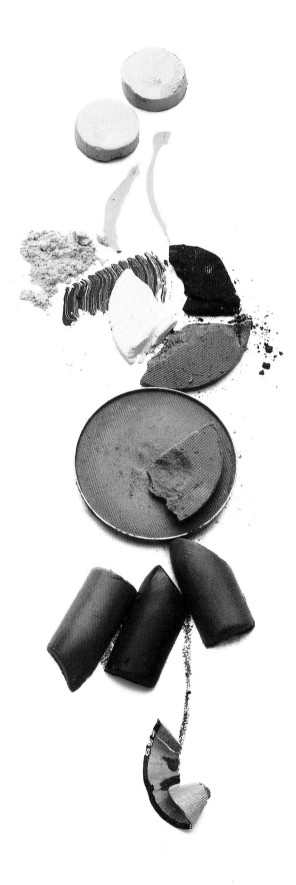

10

TEN-STEP MAKEUP APPLICATION

I have organized makeup application into ten easy steps. This is the same essential procedure I follow, whether I am making up Susan Sarandon, Christy Turlington, my mother, or myself. The basic idea is to concentrate first on achieving a smooth, even complexion (steps one, two, and three). There will be some days when concealer and powder is all you will want or need. If so, stop here. Most of the time, however, you will want to continue on to define your eyes (steps four through seven). Last comes brightening your face with cheek and lip color (steps eight through ten).

It is a good idea to follow the same basic organization every time you apply makeup. It will help you remember the steps and accomplish them more efficiently. (You'll be surprised by how quickly you can complete these steps!) If you are a real beginner, start slowly. Do only one or two steps each day until you are comfortable. Then, as you build confidence, add another step, and so on.

If you are looking for a stronger or more made-up look, choose brighter or darker tones. Or explore the à la carte menu. For a basic, polished workday look, complete all ten steps.

PRE-MAKEUP

Start with a clean face. Moisturize your entire face while it is still slightly damp.

Tip: Take a minute to brush your hair or teeth while your cream or gel absorbs.

Don't apply moisturizer directly to your eyelids (it can cause eye shadow to crease). Apply under-eye cream only if you have dry skin, so that the area remains smooth and unlined; this creates an even surface for concealer. If you have oily skin, use only a tiny bit or none at all; too much can cause makeup to slide away.

Step one: concealer

Step two: foundation

Step three: powder

Step four: eyebrows

Step five: eye shadow

Step six: eyeliner

Step seven: mascara

Step eight: blush

Step nine: lipstick
(to brighten face with color)

Step ten: lip liner

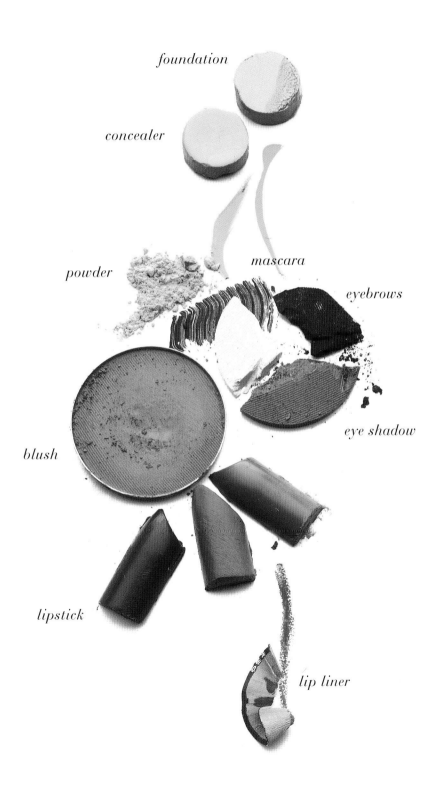

foundation

concealer

powder

mascara

eyebrows

eye shadow

blush

lipstick

lip liner

Step one: concealer

Step two: foundation
Note the three shades: light, medium, and dark

Step three: powder

Step four: eyebrows

Step five: eye shadow

Step six: eyeliner

Step seven: mascara

Step eight: blush

Step nine: lipstick
(here, a richly pigmented range of four colors)

Step ten: lip liner

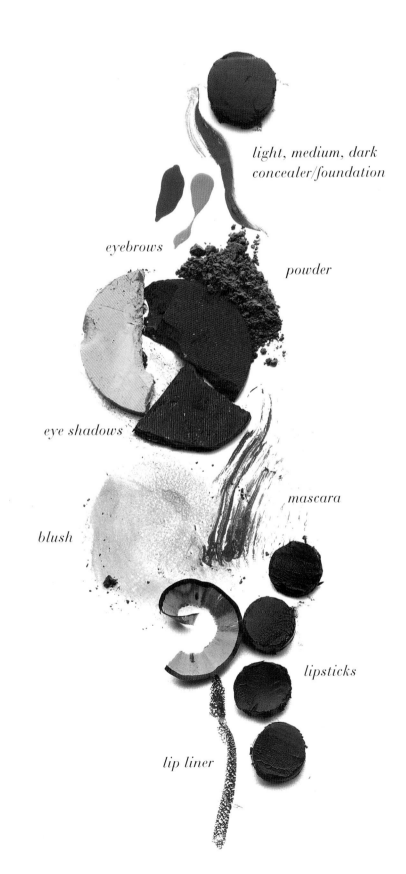

*light, medium, dark
concealer/foundation*

powder

eyebrows

eye shadows

mascara

blush

lipsticks

lip liner

À LA CARTE

Extra makeup steps for special occasions, or when you have extra time or want to try something new.

BRONZING CREAM

Use instead of foundation.

BRONZING POWDER

Dust over entire face to warm complexion.

FALSE EYELASHES

For a special party look.

SHIMMER SHADOW

Wear only a slight shimmer and choose whether to use a shimmer lid or shimmer lip—not both at the same time. Don't wear a shimmer blush—it's never flattering. Shimmer in nail enamel is fine.

LIP GLOSS

Apply with sponge applicator or your finger on top of lip color. A nice, quick touch for evening.

SHIMMER, DRAMATIC LIP COLORS

The fastest, easiest place to experiment since you can always wipe it off.

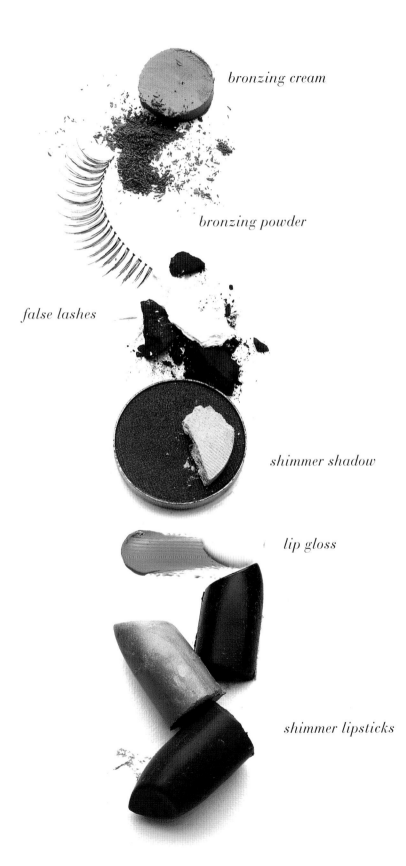

bronzing cream

bronzing powder

false lashes

shimmer shadow

lip gloss

shimmer lipsticks

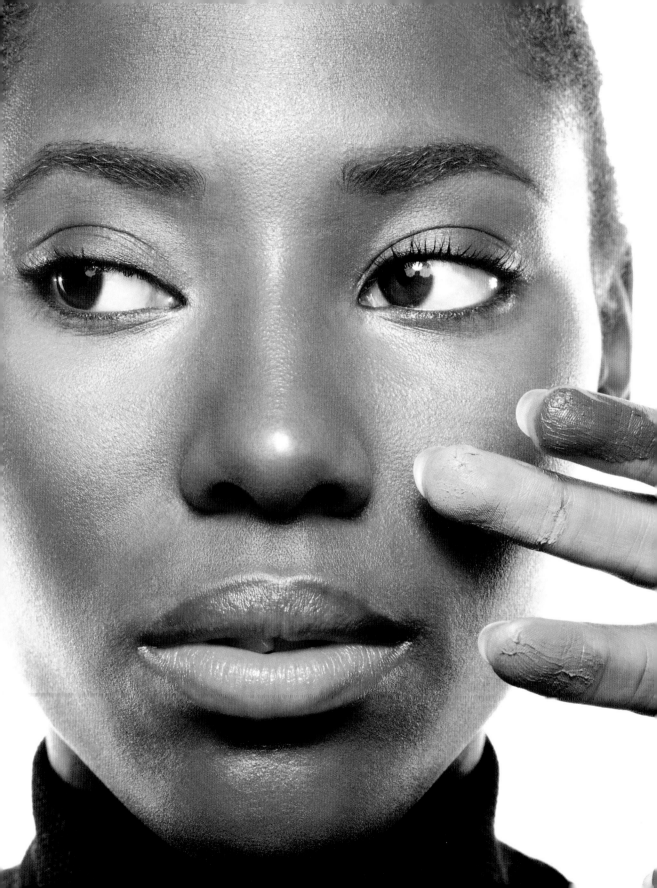

11

CONCEALERS, FOUNDATION, AND POWDER

CONCEALER

Concealer can change your life. It can make dark circles disappear. It can make you look as if you've had eight hours sleep when you've only had five. It can instantly brighten your face and lift your mood. If you have good technique and the right products, concealer can do more for your face than almost anything. It has become extremely important to me—I sometimes wear only concealer—but that has only been the case since I turned thirty. The best makeup artists are masters of concealer, often mixing their own shades. Getting concealer to work for you, however, takes a little practice.

Buying the Right Concealer

Look for a creamy texture—it should be smooth to the touch. Avoid products that feel greasy, dry, or thick or that have a chalky consistency. Concealers come in pots, sticks, or tubes with sponge applicators. I like to use stick foundation as my concealer: I like the coverage it provides, and it does not travel once I've applied it.

Finding the Right Concealer Color

The right concealer shade is yellow-based, not white, which will be much too light on the face. The biggest mistake women make with concealer is using a too light or too white shade. Search for a concealer that is one to two shades (i.e., subtly) lighter than your skin tone.

Avoid: Green-, purple-, or pink-tinted concealers, which only serve to make your face green, purple, or pink!

Applying

I recommend putting concealer under the eye up to the lower lashes and, most important, on the innermost corner of the eye. This is the most recessed area of the face and therefore the darkest-appearing. It is also a neglected spot for most women. A concealer brush is a small, firm brush that comes to a point at the tip and is especially helpful in reaching this corner. Or, as with almost any makeup application, you may use a finger to apply concealer.

Smooth and blend, using a gentle pressing action with the pads of your first two fingers. Be gentle: You don't want to end up rubbing concealer away. The aim is to make concealer as smooth as possible so that powder locks onto it in an even texture and isn't distracting or visible.

Then, *to set* the concealer, dust on yellow-toned powder using a velour puff. Use a *generous* amount, because more is better here: too much is not a problem, while too little is. Simply dust away any excess with a brush. The powder keeps the concealer *locked* in place. Moreover, the yellow tone of the powder does wonders to lighten dark circles.

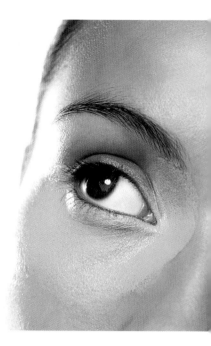

Tips

- Use your finger to blend in and smooth concealer. Make sure that you move your finger in small and gentle pats. One of the most common mistakes in applying concealer is overzealous blending. I often see women using a sweeping motion with their fingers in an attempt to blend concealer. The effect, however, is to wipe the product completely off the face.
- Never apply concealer on the eyelid; it will cause eye shadow to smear and crease.
- Many women also have redness around the base of the nose, above the upper lip, or between brows. Apply *foundation* to these areas rather than concealer. Since concealer is lighter than your skin tone, applying concealer in these areas would only draw extra attention to them. Because foundation matches the skin tone exactly, it causes these areas to blend in with the rest of your skin, becoming less obvious to the world.

Problem: Concealer makes my face look chalky.

Solution: Your concealer shade is probably too light for your skin tone. Find one that is only slightly lighter than the color of your face. Your powder may also be too white or too coarse. The worst concealer mistake is to have too white, reverse-raccoon eyes.

Problem: Concealer makes my eyes look more lined, more crepey, or, somehow, baggier.

Solution: The texture of your concealer is probably too heavy. It might be dragging your skin down. Also, if your skin is dry, you may need to apply eye cream before applying concealer. Apply only a bit and make sure it has a matte finish so that concealer will look smooth on top of it.

Note: If you have extremely oily skin, you may want to skip eye cream; it can cause concealer to travel off the eye area.

Problem: My concealer makes my mascara run below my eyes, and I hate the mess.

Solution: Pay close attention to the balance of moist surfaces (cream and concealer) with the dry ones (your own skin and powder). You are using either too much concealer and/or eye cream or too little powder. Or all three.

Problem: I put concealer on in the morning, and I like how it looks. But two hours later it's gone. What can I do?

Solution: You are not using enough concealer or enough powder. The technique that guarantees long wear is the layering of small amounts of concealer and powder. Do two to three layers for best results.

Problem: My dark circles are so permanent, I don't think anything will help.

Solution: Carry your concealer and powder in your makeup kit for reapplications throughout the day. Try a slightly brighter shade of blush or lipstick to pull attention away from your eyes. Also, open up the eye area by not wearing liner or mascara on your lower lashes.

For extremely dark circles, choose a heavy-formula concealer in a shade that is slightly lighter than your skin tone. The texture of this product will not be as smooth as a creamy concealer. But if you are really frustrated with dark circles, heavy-formula concealer is a good option.

FOUNDATION

The whole reason I wear makeup is to make my skin look smooth. For me, beauty is all about the skin. Most women, I venture to guess, probably have that same motivation. When you look at someone whom you find pretty, most likely she has clear, smooth skin. It's an essential component to good looks.

Foundation is the surest way I know to get the smooth skin I want. Some women, it seems, have bad associations with the word foundation. They fear that by wearing it, they are committing to the most grown-up, serious cosmetics artifice. They associate it with heavy, masklike makeup. They think it sounds old-fashioned, like something their mothers—or grandmothers—would do: "Foundation? Isn't that what lingerie used to be called?" Perhaps the word is unfortunate and dated. But the good it can do for you is enormous.

Foundation doesn't have to be a big commitment or an involved science. On days when I don't have much time, I may choose to use a foundation stick just to even out my spots. You will determine for yourself how much foundation to use and when. If you have never worn foundation, start with the lightest, most natural option—like a lightweight tinted face moisturizer. (There! Then you won't even have to call it foundation!)

Buying Foundation

Since this is such a key item in your makeup kit, don't scrimp here. Even if you buy all your other makeup at drugstores or discount stores, try, if at all possible, to purchase foundation at a department store. There you can get professional guidance in choosing a formula and shade, and you can test a color before buying it. The foundations sold in the higher-end make-up lines also tend to be lighter and more natural-looking.

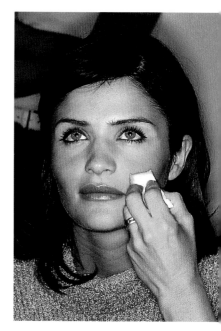

Not even the most experienced salesperson will be able to tell you which is the exact shade of foundation for you. He or she may be able to show you the closest possibilities, but you will have to take it from there. Carry a mirror with you when shopping for foundation so that you can do the natural-light foundation test. Don't let a salesperson talk you out of this exercise—it's the only thing that really works. This is a case where you must be your own makeup artist and judge the shade for yourself. In my experience, however, I find that foundation with a yellow tone looks better on almost everyone, no matter what your coloring. And almost every makeup company has at least one yellow-toned foundation in its line. Ask to see only the yellow-toned foundations and, from these options, focus on finding the best one for you.

Note: In the winter, when your skin is paler, you can mix concealer color with your foundation to lighten the foundation so it matches your skin tone.

Oily Skin: Look for an oil-free liquid foundation. Many companies offer both sheer and slightly heavier formulas. Unless you simply want to tint your face, I would recommend the slightly heavier formula, as it is better able to even out redness and blotching. Thin formulas won't give coverage no matter how much you put on.

If you choose to wear moisturizer, look for a mattifying formula—one that dries down matte, smoothing the appearance of the skin.

Normal-to-Dry Skin: Choose a creamy liquid foundation or a stick foundation. In hot, humid weather, an oil-free formula will look and feel better. (If you are worried about your skin feeling dry, use a slightly heavier moisturizer.)

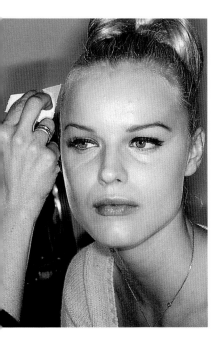

Always prime your skin with moisturizer before applying foundation and give it a minute to absorb.

To Apply

To apply foundation, use a disposable, white, triangular synthetic sponge, a fatter washable sponge, or your fingertips. Do not use a natural sea sponge; it absorbs a surprising volume of foundation and leaves nothing for your face.

Apply foundation to the center of cheeks and forehead and blend toward the edge of your face to assure even coverage. Do not apply to eyelids or under eyes when you have already applied concealer. (Foundation will negate the lightening effect of the concealer.) Start with less foundation than you think you need—it's easier to add a little more later than to remove it. Blend gently and carefully, especially around the nose and mouth.

If you feel you've put on too much or that you have created a lumpy texture, use the flats of both hands to smooth over your face, moving gently from the center toward the hairline and jawline. Use consistent pressure and a slow, smooth movement—don't tug on or rub skin. If there's still too much visible foundation, use a tissue to lift off the excess. Again, don't rub or else everything will come off.

To set the foundation, take a velour powder puff and use it to press powder over the foundation; this locks the foundation into place and helps prevent oil breakthrough. Dust off excess powder with powder brush.

You don't need to use foundation all over your face; you can also dot it on trouble spots, then blend.

To conceal blemishes, apply foundation using a concealer brush. Do not use concealer; since it is lighter than your skin tone, it will only draw light and attention to the area. Because your foundation matches your skin tone, anything it covers should disappear. Foundation is also moisturizing, which makes for a smoother, creamier finish. Remember to use powder to lock in foundation.

Tips

- Shake foundation bottle vigorously before applying. Even though foundations should not noticeably separate, the heavier parts do tend to drop to the bottom of the container.
- Avoid two-phase foundation formulas (they usually have a watery liquid phase on top of the bottle and a heavier liquid phase underneath),

which are sometimes designed for acne-prone skin. I find that they make skin look rough and chalky. Also, avoid dual-finish foundations: They create a rough surface and can look fake.

• Note that most of the more recent oil free foundations that have come on the market contain one or more silicone-based ingredients. The result is formulas that are extremely light and have much more slip to the feel. Decide for yourself whether you like the touch.

Question: What can I use to even out my skin tone if I don't like the feel of foundation?

Answer: Spot-apply foundation only on uneven areas and around the nose, which tends to be red. Use a warm-tinted powder (not translucent powder) with a puff to set foundation and create a more natural finish.

Question: I have a yellow skin tone. Should I use makeup that's yellow or counter my skin tone with another shade?

Answer: The only appropriate foundation to wear is one that disappears on your face, which means finding a foundation that is yellow in tone. Then you may choose to use pink or rosy blush to counter your skin tone.

Question: I have fair skin and red hair. Should I really be wearing a yellow-toned foundation?

Answer: Even the palest ivory foundation should have a yellow undertone to look natural. Pale yellow foundation works to warm a very fair complexion. If a product contains too much yellow, however, it will appear too dark on your skin.

BOBBI'S FOUNDATION TEST

Finding the perfect foundation is the number one, most important thing in the makeup world. The right foundation should not be heavy or artificial. It should, in fact, be so perfectly matched to your skin tone and texture that it disappears. You see not makeup but smooth, flawless skin.

If you already own and use foundation, try this test: Apply a swipe of it on your cheek. Then grab a small mirror and step outside into completely natural light. Look to see if the foundation is visible. If it's very hard to see on your face, your foundation works. If the swipe is obvious and visible, it's time to get a new foundation.

BOBBI'S COLOR PRINCIPLE

Every woman should own three tones of concealer/foundation. Many black women use three tones on a daily basis to even out varying skin tones.

Light: Everyday concealer color. Note: When you have a tan, switch to medium tone as concealer and dark tone as foundation.

Medium: Your basic everyday foundation.

Dark: Summer foundation, or whenever you have a tan.

The idea is to mix any combination of the three anytime you need and to monitor periodically the exact match of color. That way you will avoid multiple jar purchases in search of the "perfect" shade.

Note: It is important to check your skin tone periodically; the foundation that disappeared on your face (i.e., was perfectly matched) six months ago may be too light or too dark today because of a normal change in skin tone due to seasonal changes.

POWDER

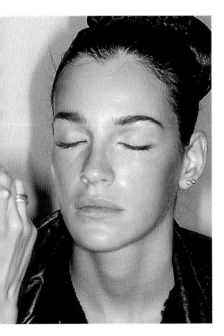

Powder is one of the makeup essentials that you'll want to get right. Wearing the correct powder will give your face a smooth appearance. It will hold your concealer and foundation in place. The right powder has the power to save a foundation that is slightly too dark or too pale. (Pale yellow powder can sometimes even make a too pink foundation look good.) And, most important, the right powder should be practically invisible.

The wrong powder is chalky and heavy, and can look horrible. That may explain why many women cringe when I mention powder. Some women would like to skip the whole category of powder. But that would be a mistake: Powder is absolutely essential to keeping makeup on your face.

My powder philosophy is one of the things that defines me as a makeup artist. I believe that the most magical, universal, and workable powder for all skin colors is pale yellow in tone. If I could convert all women to this one tenet of beauty, I would be thrilled! I am just as adamant that translucent powder is not the way to go. Translucent powders are not translucent at all: They create a chalky, pale effect that is quite visible and most unattractive to the eye.

Powder Texture

Powder should feel silky and smooth in your hand. It should seem like it is lighter than air. You are the best judge, so feel for yourself.

Powder Shade

Ninety-five (or even ninety-eight or ninety-nine) percent of the time, I find that a yellow-toned powder is much more flattering to a woman's face than pink powders or so-called flesh-toned powders. This is because almost all women have yellow tones to their skin. Yellow-toned powders have a magical effect on the face, warming it and equalizing its hue with that of your hands, chest, arms, etc. The idea of yellow powder in your cosmetic bag may be strange at first. But try it and see for yourself what it does for your face.

I especially do *not* recommend translucent powder. Many women think it's invisible, but it's not. On the contrary, I find that translucent powder makes a woman look pasty. Pale yellow is the only powder shade that truly lightens dark circles.

There are many other powder colors on the market that promise to even out skin tone. The theory behind purple, pink, or green powder is that it will "correct" complementary, unattractive color in the face. My advice is: Don't bother. These powders are pretty to look at, but they do not work.

Dark pressed powders are excellent for contouring bronzer, as they tend to be sheer and easy to blend. Dark powder is also an excellent way to counter a too light foundation.

Loose v. Pressed

Loose powder is your at-home, stationary powder. It provides more coverage than pressed powder, especially if used with a velour powder puff, and is quite economical.

Since loose powder can get messy in transit and is bulky, pressed powder is the mobile powder—the one to take with you during the day for touch-ups and when you are on the road.

Your pressed-powder compact is probably one of the only makeup items you'll use in public, so choose a compact you really like. There are endless varieties—from vintage silver or gold to fancy jeweled compacts to modern brushed–stainless steel and plain matte black.

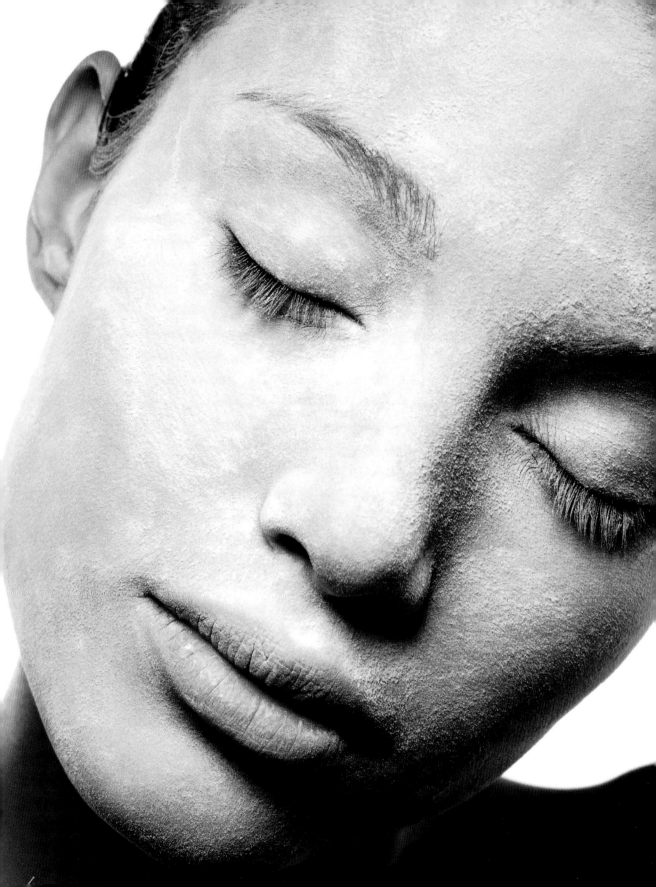

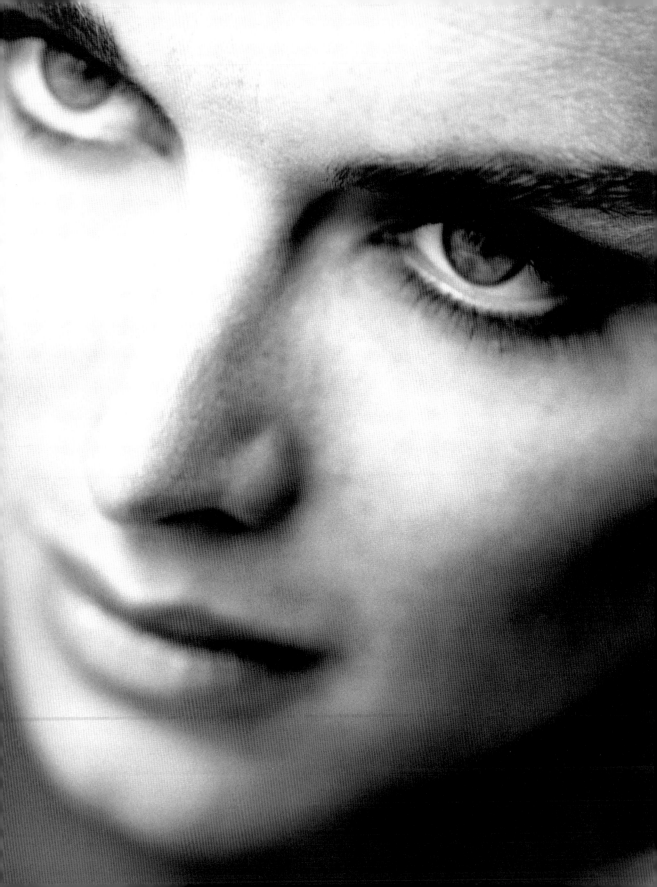

12

BROWS: SHAPING, GROOMING, AND DEFINING

The brow is the face's forgotten feature. Through the ages, poets and musicians have extolled mysterious eyes, sensual lips, satiny skin, and extraordinary hair. But eyebrows? Nonetheless, a well-groomed, well-defined brow can be extremely flattering and add considerable strength to a woman's eyes. It can open up her face so that she actually needs less makeup. A well-shaped brow can also help lift deep-set eyes or maximize small eyes. There are even instances where a lifted, well-manicured brow has had the same effect as a surgical eye-lift.

In evolutionary terms, the brow is the face's own protection. Like eyelashes, the brow is meant to keep foreign objects out of the eyes. So there is a good, natural reason not to take too much of it away.

BROW SHAPE

You are born with a brow shape that works naturally with your eyes and face. Your brow's own natural line should be your guide. I strongly discourage women from severe plucking, because, unlike eyelashes, brow hairs do not always grow completely back.

Like every other aspect of makeup, brow styles come and go. In the 1940s, women shaved their brows and then painted on thin black lines. In the early 1960s, a narrow brow line was again the fashion, but it was achieved through exaggerated plucking. Thanks to Brooke Shields and Margaux Hemingway, a stronger, androgynous brow phase took hold in the late 1970s. That was a big moment for brows. Since then, brow style has been generally more manicured. But, strange as it sounds, brow fashion today changes slightly almost every season. Models sometimes have a hard time keeping up. Many who have allowed their brows to be radically plucked take isolated, lengthy vacations for the unsightly growing-back phase. In some cases, eyebrows never come back quite the same.

GENERAL BROW PRINCIPLE

Eyebrows have to work with your features and style. If you are small or have delicate features, your brow should have a finer line (think Michelle Pfeiffer or Linda Evangelista).

Conversely, if you have an athletic build and a healthy, natural look, your brow should probably be a little thicker and less manicured. Clean up only between the brows and under the arch (as in Brooke Shields or Christy Turlington).

If you have small, deep-set eyes, you have the most to gain from a well-shaped brow. A well-defined brow creates a strong eye statement without the use of dark eye colors, which, by the way, can make a small eye look even smaller (think Demi Moore, Jodie Foster, or me!).

Once you begin to focus on the brow it can become an obsession. And once you change the shape of your brow through plucking, plan to maintain it with weekly or biweekly cleanups.

HOW TO PLUCK

Unless you really know what you are doing, plucking can be frustrating. If you feel agitated, you may end up doing too drastic a job. Try not to be hasty or in a rush. It's best to start slowly and do only one clear task. Wait a day or a two before picking up the tweezers again.

Start by removing only the hairs that appear above your nose, between the two brows. The beginning of your brow should be even with the inside corner of your eye. Stop and, if necessary, pluck again another day.

Next, remove any obviously stray hairs below your brow. A nicely opened eye area is one of the effects of a well-groomed brow. The rule along the length of the brow is to pluck only from beneath the brow.

Then clean up the shape, making sure that the arch of the brow occurs three-quarters of the way out. Let the brow extend beyond the outside corner of your eye. At that point, it should taper slightly down. When plucking from the body of the brow, check along the length of each individual hair to see where its root falls. Make sure you will not be creating a hole by removing it.

Note: If you have long brow hairs, trim them with manicure scissors to keep them looking neat. It's a good idea to trim before you tweeze; it will help you see the natural shape of your brow and locate where individual hairs fall.

TIPS

- Invest in good tweezers (Tweezerman is one quality brand), ideally with a flat, slanted tip. As long as you don't lose them, you'll never have to buy another.
- Pluck brows in a room with plentiful daylight.
- It is much less painful to pluck brows just after a shower, when pores are still open. (Some women use Anbesol to numb the area before plucking. Others recommend icing the brow to cut the pain, but I have never found that to help; besides, it's messy.)

PROFESSIONAL BROW HELP

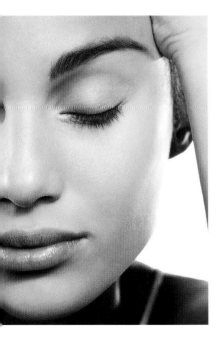

It is very difficult to shape your own brow correctly. It is equally difficult to find someone who can do a good job of it for you. The best solution, I find, to locating the best brow waxer, hairstylist, trainer, or masseuse is to be a beauty networker; talk to your friends and work associates. Ask around to learn which salons in your community do waxing. Be sure to note the name of the person who performs the service as well. Don't be too fazed by the elegance (or nonelegance) of the salon since, basically, the waxing will be only as good as the person doing it.

The one possible drawback to brow waxing is in-grown hairs, which can be quite painful and unsightly. To avoid them, clean the brow area with a toner immediately after waxing. Exfoliate with a gentle, grainy scrub regularly so that hairs will not get trapped beneath the skin.

Professional tweezing is probably the best option, but it is offered much less frequently than waxing. Ask around for makeup artists and salon aestheticians who do this service. A semiannual waxing or tweezing appointment may be all you need: Once you establish the correct shape, upkeep—as long as you tweeze weekly or biweekly—is relatively easy.

Tinting is another salon option that is relatively fast and inexpensive. It is especially nice for blond brows that are so light they disappear. In that case, I recommend going a shade or two darker than your hair color. (If you feel discomfort in your eyes when the tint is applied, stop the process. You are probably allergic.) Never tint your brows black, even if your hair is naturally black or dyed black. The result is much too harsh; your brows look almost painted on. Try brown tones instead. If your hair contains any red highlights, try mahogany tones.

BROW MISTAKES

Paisley-Shaped Brows: A common tweezing mistake. Shaping the brow so that it has a round clump or hook at the inner end and then trails off narrowly never looks good.

Excessive Tweezing, Holes: Overaggressive tweezing will result in bare spots, or holes, in the line of the brow. Try to see where a hair falls and what the overall picture will be before tugging away.

Tattooing: I am totally against tattooing the brow; it never looks natural. It is much too extreme a measure.

Shaving: Even if you really hate your eyebrows, shaving them off is not the solution. With repeated shaving over the years, brows do not grow back fully or regularly.

No Maintenance: Every adult woman should do a basic brow cleanup no matter how natural her look.

MAKING UP BROWS

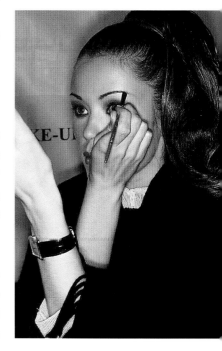

Filling in the brow is an essential makeup step. Since its effect can be huge—framing your face and giving it strength—it should be as automatic as coating on mascara. I think a lot of women skip the brow because they never step back from the mirror to see themselves from a distance—the way most people view you. (Looking at oneself too closely in the mirror might also explain our obsession with mascara.) Making up the brow is always one of my top three makeup steps.

Many women have had bad experiences trying to use brow pencils, hating that their brows looked too dark and unnatural. Using eye shadow as a filler, however, has a much more natural effect. Do your brows as detailed below, then take a few steps back from the mirror. It should be clear to you now how the brow can define the face without looking painted on. This is especially true for Asian women and blond and/or fair-skinned women. In making up the brow, Asian women should focus on creating a thicker line.

I almost always use shadow to fill in the brow. My rule of thumb for shadow color is brown. Anything too yellow or too black ends up looking unnatural. If you prefer a brow pencil, find one that is very soft to avoid looking artificial.

If hair color is:	Use shadow brow filler in:
blond	taupe
light brown	sable
red	taupe or camel
brunette with red highlights	red brown
true brown	mahogany
black	the darkest brown, never charcoal or black
gray	slate or gray

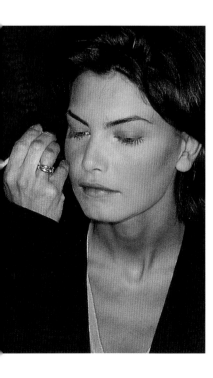

To apply, use a small, hard brush, flat and angled at the tip. For longer-lasting color, dampen the brush slightly before dipping it into the shadow color. Blow off the excess and start applying it at the most populated area of brow to avoid laying down too much color. Finish by combing your brows up with a hard eyebrow brush or a firm toothbrush that you've designated for the job.

TIPS

To tone down a too dark or too heavy brow color application, press face powder onto your brow with a powder puff.

- For holes in your brow, fill in with brow pencil. Then go over entire length of brow with shadow, using a brush.
- To create a brow where hair is sparse or nonexistent, use a brow pencil to draw in the brow line. Then go over the line with shadow, using a brush.
- To lengthen brows that are too short, use the above technique—pencil first, then shadow.
- Brown mascara may also be used to fill in brow. But this requires a light touch—if there's too much mascara on the wand, wipe it down with a tissue.

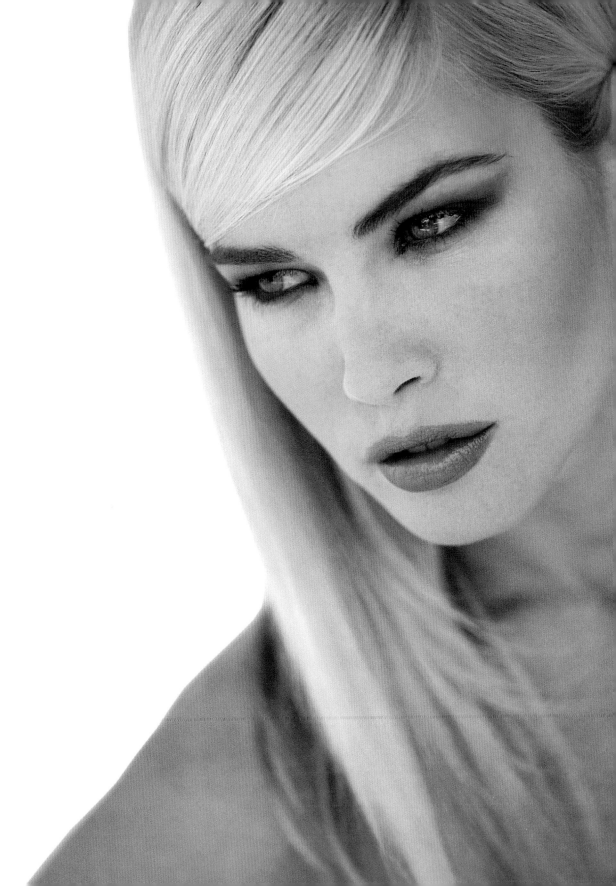

13

EYE ESSENTIALS: SHADOW, LINER, AND MASCARA

EYE SHADOW

In developing my color palette for the eyes, I have purposely avoided colors like emerald green, turquoise, and purple. That's because I would much rather let a woman's own eye color pop than make a bold statement with the shadow shade. I have also avoided trendy shadow colors—the pale blue you see in fashion magazines this month will be out of style by the time you buy and wear it.

The following chart represents a series of suggestions for shadow combinations, based on skin and hair coloring. The basic idea is to choose complementary colors in three intensities, light (for highlighting), medium (for lower half of lid), and dark (to be used at lash line as liner). While you need not necessarily buy these exact colors, it is important to stay within the same color range. Colors worn on the lid should blend naturally together so that there are not three separate swipes of shadow. Highlighter should be a natural extension of the shadow and the liner shades, perhaps even a less intense version of the others. What doesn't work? Mixing pink highlighter, moss shadow, and navy liner; these colors do not blend well together. (Wear gray shadow instead, however, and it works nicely!)

	Highlighter	Shadow	Liner
Fair Hair,	bone	taupe	cocoa/sable
Light Skin	white	gray	slate/navy
	bone	heather	dark brown
Brown Hair,	bone	sable	mahogany
Medium Skin	banana	cocoa	navy
	pale pink	slate	charcoal
Dark Hair,	banana	cocoa	mahogany
Dark Skin	toast	sable	mahogany
	pale pink	slate	charcoal

Pre-Makeup Warning: Avoid putting anything creamy on your eyelids (moisturizer, foundation, or concealer); it will crease or cake your eye shadow.

TO APPLY

Prime the eye, using a velour powder puff to dust your eyelid with face powder. Then, using a shadow brush, apply your highlighter shadow all over lid, from lash line to brow.

Apply medium shadow color on your lower lid, from lash line to the crease of your eye.

Use the darkest shadow color as liner. Dampen a narrow eyeliner brush before applying any shadow; this will make for longer wear. Make an X in your eye shadow with your dampened brush and then drag only the tip of the brush through the X you've created; following this pattern will help ensure that you are picking up a sufficient amount of powder. Blow off any excess powder; this will ensure that your shadow will not flake.

Grasp the liner brush as you would a normal writing pencil, and place it close to your eye. Lift your chin and tilt your head back slightly as you look in the mirror, so that you can see clearly along your lash line. Be careful to line the full length of the eye: Don't forget the space between the inner corner of the eye and the beginning of the lashes. If you have light-colored lashes, be especially careful to apply liner on top of lashes so that there is no blank space between lash and lid.

Contour shadow as desired for evening or special events. Use a medium-tone shadow with a contour brush. Apply at the outer corner of eye, following the natural line of the brow bone. (See Special Effect Contouring below.)

To apply mascara, roll the wand as you stroke mascara on your lashes. Rather than piling on a lot of mascara in one coat, do two or three light coats, waiting briefly between coats to allow mascara to dry.

Finally, add a touch of highlighting color. Use your finger or shadow brush to place a little highlighter just below the most arched portion of the brow.

Shadow Tips

- In general, it is fresher to have light colors on the lid rather than dark. Light colors open up the eyes rather than make them seem to recede.

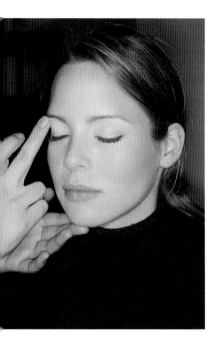

It's a basic makeup principle: Light stands out, dark recedes. (The same applies to concealer, which is used to lighten dark, recessed areas.)

- To find the most natural-looking shadow colors, examine the colors that occur naturally on your eyelid and match them with sheer shadow shades.
- The most fundamental lesson about eye color is to use colors that blend together naturally. The trick is not where you put the color—it should never be apparent that there are three different colors. The shades should work together naturally and blend together invisibly.
- Do not rub eye shadow with your fingertips in an attempt to blend or soften colors—this will simply remove all the color or transfer the make-up onto your clothes. Wiping away color is a natural impulse when things look too intense—but resist. Instead, use a powder puff with face powder and press it on your eyelid to tone down shadow color.
- Using shadow along the lash line creates a softer line than pencil liner and is easier to control.

The Most Common Eye Makeup Mistakes

Cat Eyes: Black liquid liner that extends upward—well beyond the outside corner of the eye—is harsh and looks dated. Brown shadow liner drawn a tiny bit past the eye is softer.

Kaleidoscope Eyes: Bright, shocking mismatched colors don't belong on the eyelid (unless you are dressing as a clown for Halloween!). Choose muted colors in the same family and blend them well.

Blush as Shadow: Sweeping your blush color across your lid sounds like a useful time-saver (lots of makeup artists make just this suggestion). I find that the rosy coloration of most blushes are wrong for the eye area and can cause eyes to appear red or pink. Do the same one-color technique with shadow shades like toast or pale pink.

Unfinished Liner: Lining only the outside half of the eye has a minimizing effect. You may choose to do only the top lid, but be sure to apply color all the way from the inside corner of eye, continue along the entire lash line to the outermost corner.

Shadow Matching: It's almost never a good idea to match your eye shadow color to your eye color—especially if you have blue or green eyes. Blue eyes look amazing with navy liner but disappear with blue shadow. In general, neutral colors that contrast with eye color work better.

Mascara Clumps: It was the look in the 1960s, but it doesn't work today. The best way to achieve thick, thick lashes is to do several thin coats of mascara. If you experience clumping, wipe the excess mascara from your brush with a tissue.

Question: I sometimes have droopy eyes when I am tired. How should I make them up?

Answer: The more tired you are, the less eye makeup you should use.

Try dusting your light-to-medium shadow shade all over the eyelid. Do a light application of mascara on upper lashes only.

LINER

Liner is a magnet for attention. It draws attention to the eyes and forces eye contact—even from strangers. (I definitely get noticed more when I wear liner.) Even if you have deep-set eyes, liner will make your eyes stand out, maximizing them.

If you have blue eyes, your eye color will be best accented by brown or navy liner. I also like charcoal for night.

If you have brown eyes, use dark brown or cocoa liner.

If you have green eyes, try brown shadow. Or, if there's a yellow undertone to your eyes, camel or pale yellow shadow is the best complement.

Liner Don'ts

Never apply liner to the inside rim of your eye. Ophthalmologists universally admonish women (and makeup artists) not to use this technique.

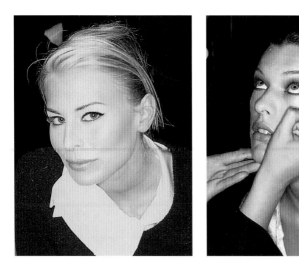

Applying liner so close to the eye surface increases the risk of injuring the eye. In addition, there is the risk of infection to the eye from the eyeliner, which seeps easily onto the eye surface, and from the brush surface, especially if it has not recently been cleaned.

Aesthetically, wearing liner on the rim of the eye doesn't work. By lining so close to the eye, you make it look smaller. It is very high-maintenance as well, as you must constantly wipe away the residue from the inner corner of eye.

White eyeliner applied to the rim of the eye looks like, well, white liner applied to the rim of the eye. It doesn't magically make eyes look gigantic. (This is, however, a regular part of stage makeup.)

SPECIAL EFFECT CONTOURING: RX FOR PUFFY EYES AND RECEDING LIDS

I really do not like the word contouring, because it implies changing the shape of a feature. I do, however, like one specific contouring technique that gives strength to the eye and definition for women with puffy eyes or receding lids.

Use your medium shadow (or one shade darker) with a contour brush. The idea is to apply a sideways V shape at the outside third of your eye; it will frame your eye nicely. It involves two strokes: The top stroke should start at the upper outside corner of eye and work the shadow inward, down toward eye crease. The second stroke should start at outside lower corner of eye at the lash line—work shadow inward and up to crease, meeting the other line. Pat the shadow with finger to soften edges.

To contour for day, use this same technique, but choose a soft color that doesn't need blending. Try a deeper color for night or for a special event.

MASCARA

In terms of makeup loyalty, mascara rates number one. It seems that once a woman finds a mascara that she loves, she is apt to buy it again and again. Mascara is also very high on the list of makeup products women say they can't leave home without. It is among the first cosmetic items young women buy for themselves. Mascara is sort of like laundry detergent: Women figure out what they like and then are loathe to change.

Mascara has never been a hotbed of experimentation—even when it comes to color. In a word, most women wear black. I agree—I like black mascara best, too. Some women like brown-black as a casual-day option. But brown-black is so close to black that you might as well stick to black. Brown mascara gives the most natural, un-made-up eye. If you have blond lashes (often the case with strawberry blondes), reddish brown mascara is the prettiest option. Avoid navy, purple, or red mascaras—they almost never look good.

TIPS

- If your mascara is too gooey or wet, use a tissue to blot lashes after coating on.
- I find that I get good lash separation if I roll the wand as I am combing it through the lashes.
- Always apply mascara to the upper lashes from underneath and to the lower lashes from on top. (Putting mascara on the top of upper lashes looks heavy and gloppy.)
- Always use less mascara on your lower lashes.
- For a cleaner, more open look to your face, try skipping your lower lashes altogether. (Remember this option for a day when you are tired-looking or pressed for time.)
- Always apply mascara with the wand held parallel to the floor. Never point the tip of the mascara into your eye. It causes clumps and is quite dangerous.
- Never apply mascara in a moving vehicle.

MASCARA 101

Waterproof Mascara: A good idea if you are going to be filmed for video or television, play sports, or plan to cry at a function. Always wear waterproof mascara to weddings, especially your own. I don't recommend it for daily use, however, since it can be drying to the lashes. Apply two to three fine, thin coats.

Brown Mascara: A really nice extra to have in your makeup kit for minimal makeup days. It creates a gentle, soft look. (If you wipe down the wand, brown mascara also works as a brow filler for blondes and brunettes.)

Thickening Mascara v. Lengthening Mascara: I prefer lengthening formulas since most go on more evenly and look more natural. Clumping occurs more often with thickening mascaras. (The remedy for clumping is to take a tissue and wipe down the mascara wand before applying—but a better alternative is to use a thinner formula.)

Navy and Other Brightly Colored Mascaras: I don't recommend using these.

Curling Lashes

If you ask the question "Do I need to curl my lashes?" the answer is probably no. You are probably lucky enough to have a natural lift to your lashes. Just for fun, though, you may want to try curling your lashes for a special occasion.

If, however, you have straight lashes, curling may be a daily necessity to open up your eyes.

To curl your lashes, look straight into the mirror and press firmly down on lash curler for five to ten seconds. Roll curler slightly up and away while holding. Then repeat on other eye.

Always curl lashes before you apply mascara; otherwise, you risk damaging or breaking lashes.

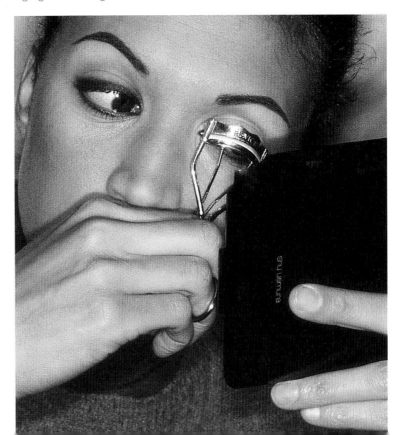

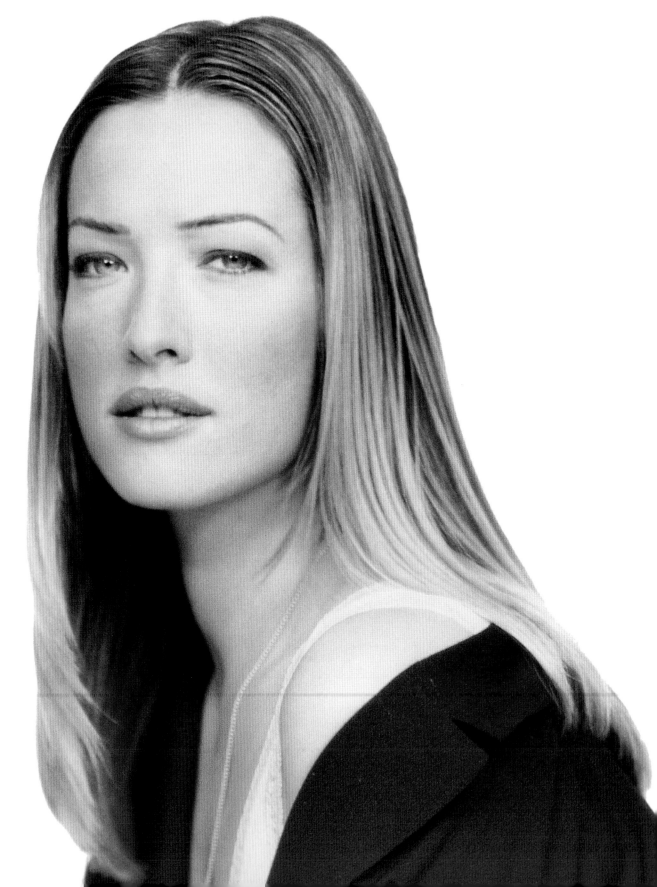

14

ALL ABOUT BLUSH

I drive people crazy with blush: Applying it to others' faces is almost an involuntary impulse for me. When I walk into a department store where I have a makeup counter, I almost always reach for blush and a brush to give a lift to the sales associates there. Nothing makes a woman look prettier than a shot of blush. And there is no faster "up" if you're lagging in the middle of a long afternoon.

While choosing the right shade of blush seems to be difficult for many women, getting it right is surprisingly simple. (And, like much of my method, you will learn to be the best judge of the blush shade that works for you.)

Your perfect blush shade is the color of your cheek when you are flushed or exercising. That is the most critical aspect of blush. Since I like blush to look natural, I prefer shades that are rose-toned, pink-toned, or tawny brown. It follows that the lighter your skin is, the lighter your blush shade should be. The darker your skin, the deeper the blush.

Matching blush tone with lipstick color might sound like advice from your grandmother, but this is one beauty rule that is well worth following. (It was once commonplace for a woman to rub a little lipstick onto her cheeks for a lift of color—the original perfect match.)

If lipstick color is:	Use this color blush:
red	reddish or pink
rose	rose
pink	pink-toned
coral or orange	peach or apricot
bronze	bronze
brown	pink, orange, or red, depending on the undertone of the lipstick

TEXTURES

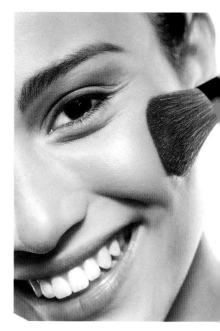

Cream Blush is preferred by a lot of older women who feel that their skin is dry and could benefit from a richer formula. For longer wear, apply cream blush, then dust with face powder and apply another pop of powder blush on top. **Gel Blush** is a nice option for smooth, young skin, since it is practically see-through.

Note: Wash your hands immediately after applying, as gel blush can stain your fingertips.

Powder Blush is the most popular choice. I recommend having two different tones in your kit—one natural shade and a second that is slightly more colorful. For all-day blush, apply the natural blush first, then dust over it with a pop of the second blush to keep the color going. Don't use the brighter blush without first applying the more muted blush base for daytime wear, since it will look too harsh. A brighter application is fine for nighttime wear, however.

To Apply

The brush that comes with most blush compacts should be discarded. It's too skinny to allow an even sweep of color. Instead, use a separate blush brush that is full and tapered at the sides. (See chapter 9.)

There are two key phrases I use over and over when I talk about blush:

• apple of cheek: area of the face where you should be applying your blush. To find your cheek's apple, smile in an exaggerated way; the fleshy, lifted part of your cheek is the most natural place to put blush.

• pop of color: a second coat of a brighter blush.

Use your blush brush both to apply and to blend your powder blush. (This is one instance when you should not use your hands to apply makeup; you risk removing most of the powder you've applied.) Dip brush into powder blush; blow off excess before you start. Apply blush first to the apple of your cheek. Blend up and back toward your hairline, but also blend down, away from your cheek-bone for a more natural look.

If you have very high cheekbones, focus blush on the center of your face, closer to your nose. Conversely, if your face is wide or full, concentrate blush closer to your hairline, away from the center of your face.

Classic Blush Mistakes

- Using shades that are too bright, too dark, or too pale.
- Blush applied in a horizontal stripe across the cheeks.
- Blush that clashes with lips, like bronze-toned blush worn with red lips.
- Blush that is too shimmery or frosted.
- Dual-finish blushes (i.e., cream/powder formulas); they can be quite heavy and create a lumpy texture on the face.

BRONZING POWDER

We've all been warned and, intellectually at least, we know that tanning is taboo; the sun is lethal. No matter. A "sun-kissed" look is still irresistible to our eyes. Happily, we have bronzing powder, which can make us look healthier and more rested instantly. Perhaps a pasty face represents zero sun damage, but it certainly doesn't make you feel very good.

I like to think of bronzing powder as a tint of overall color. It should be applied anywhere the sun naturally hits, i.e., the raised areas of your face, such as the crest of your nose, your cheekbones, and brow bones. It works great on a day when you choose not to wear a lot of foundation.

If you have dark skin, bronzing powder may be used as a natural-looking blush. (After the bronzing powder, I like to add a touch of pink or rosy blush on the apples of the cheeks.)

Avoid bronzers that are orange-toned or frosted, since they will look too artificial on your face. Most companies offer light, medium, and dark bronzers. You may find that you wear one shade in the winter and a slightly darker one in the summer. Select according to the season.

To Apply

Apply bronzing powder with a short, fluffy brush. Sweep it over the apples of your cheeks, your forehead, down the line of your nose, and on your neck (if needed to avoid an obvious makeup line). It is best applied sheer.

If you have smooth, dry skin, consider using bronzing sticks or creams. Buy the sheerest formula available and apply it with your fingers or a sponge. This will create the ultimate natural glow.

Beware: Oily skin has been known to turn bronzers an unpleasant shade of orange. If your skin is quite oily, you may have to forgo the pleasure. Instead, use a true brown pressed powder that has no orange present.

Question: What do I do if I don't have cheekbones?

Answer: This is a question I am asked quite often and it always makes me smile. I always want to respond: "Of course you have cheekbones." Everyone does.

Perhaps the more accurate way to word the question is "What do I do with my round face?"

Well, the first thing to know is that you shouldn't try to paint on cheekbones. Use blush to give your face a lift and to add a little color, but don't waste your time trying to contour in chiseled cheekbones.

The second thing to remember is that you are in very good company. Actresses Andie MacDowell and Isabella Rossellini both have quite round faces and undefined cheekbones, and both have had major cosmetics-company contracts and serious film careers. Because of their fuller face shape, these women will look forever young. So if you share this quality with them, be happy. They are two of the most beautiful women in the world!

Question: Where do I put blush so that it looks natural?

Answer: One of the biggest mistakes women make with blush is sucking in their cheeks, then applying one stripe of color across the hollow part of their faces. The result always looks artificial. (Who's idea was that, anyway?) Instead, blush should be applied on the apple of your cheek, which is where color would rise naturally if you were embarrassed, exhausted, or flushed. To find that spot, smile in an exaggerated way. The apple is the round, lifted part of your face. Also, be careful to blend blush up into your hairline.

If you have trouble blending, the problem may be your blush shade. Try buying a lighter, more neutral blush. The right color blush should almost blend itself.

Don't worry if the color seems too dull in the compact—you need a muted base to look natural. Remember that natural color is the right color, not washed-out color! You may layer a slightly brighter blush on top for a pop of color. For day, be sure to balance base blush color with color pop. At night, use your brighter blush for the perfect amount of color.

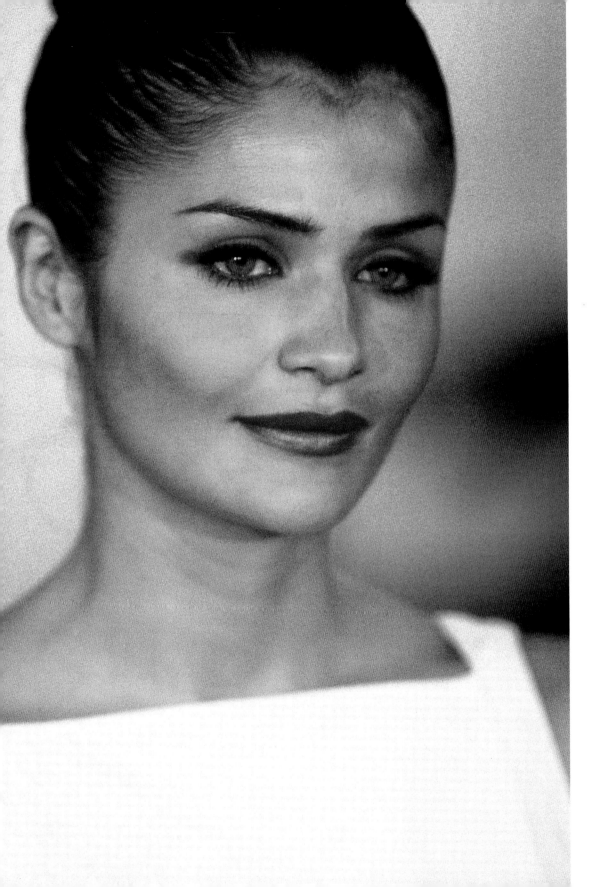

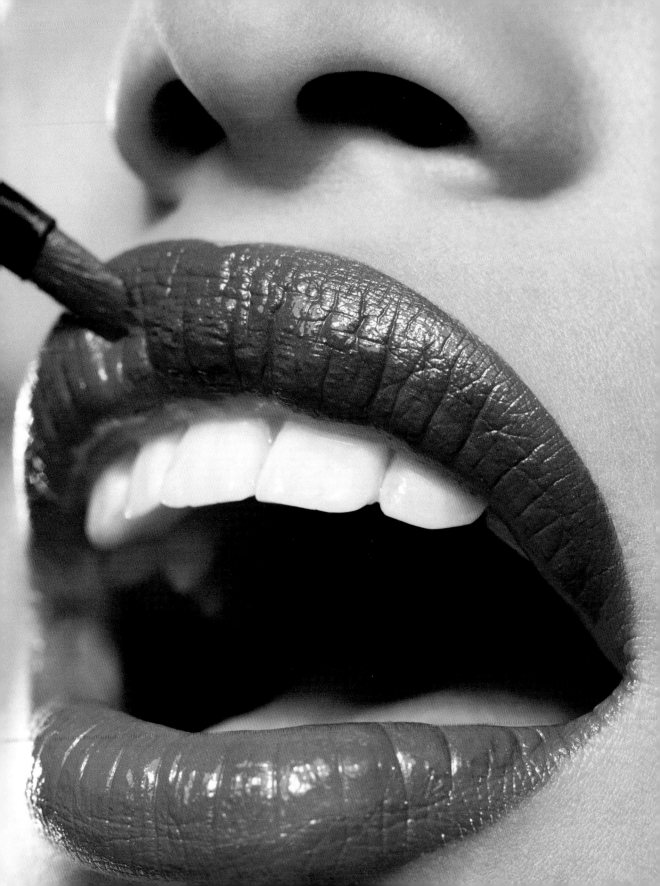

15

DOING YOUR LIPS: COLOR, FORMS AND FINISHES, TECHNIQUE

If eyes are windows of the soul, lips are the mirrors of our mood. Changing lip color is the quickest way to change your entire look. One swipe of lipstick can instantly make a woman look sexier, sweeter, bolder, more rested, more polished, more glamorous, or more put-together, depending on the color and texture chosen. Lip color can define you or change you. Lipstick can be played with, mixed, and blended, quickly and easily. (Blotting off the old color takes only a few seconds and a tissue.) You don't have to be a technical wizard to wear lipstick properly, so it's a great place to experiment and have fun with zero frustration. Lipstick is the first thing a young girl reaches for when she starts playacting with her mother's makeup. It's no wonder—the attraction is powerful.

The Search for the Perfect Lip Color

If I had to teach someone just one thing about lip color it would be this: Find a lipstick that looks good on your face when you are wearing absolutely no makeup. This is the magic color that will make your skin, hair, and eyes look their best. By definition, it will be a lip-toned color—somewhere in the range of brown-pink, nude, beige-pink, or rosy brown. When you have found it, you will know.

Balancing Act: Eye v. Lip

One of the hallmarks of modern, polished makeup is the proper balance between the eye and the lip. Both features may be made-up, but they should never compete for attention. A heavy, smoky eye calls for a neutral lip. Similarly, a big statement lip—whether red, bright, or dark—works best with a more neutral eye.

FORMS AND FINISHES

Matte Lipstick: A sophisticated option. Look for a creamy matte texture, as some matte formulas are very dry and cause lips to appear cracked and dehydrated. The only way to know if a particular brand is dry is to try it.

Note: Some women, especially those with dry skin, find that they can wear matte lip color only during the summer, when warm, humid weather melts and moistens even the most matte lipsticks.

Sheer Lipstick: An easy way to wear color. A transparent stain.

Shimmer or Frost Lipstick: I prefer shimmer (which has less mica pigments that cause the reflected effect) over frost (which has more mica pigments and is much drier).

Gloss: This is a useful option to have in your lipstick wardrobe, although it seems to go in and out of style rather frequently. Gloss is often a teen-ager's first form of lip color, but it can also be very flattering on an older woman's face because it draws light to the face and creates the appearance of fuller lips. It's usually sold in a small pot and smoothed on with the fingers.

Long-Wear Lip Color: These are newer lipsticks that promise to last as long as eight or twelve hours. As of yet I have not seen a long-lasting formula I really like: They tend to be very dry and unnatural-looking. I happen to like the look of lipstick that fades over the course of a few hours to a really pretty stain. And I don't know a man who really likes to kiss a woman wearing lipstick. Lipstick isn't meant to last forever!

Pencils: Narrow lip pencils can be used to line the lip or to color in all over, before or after applying gloss. Fatter lip pencils tend to be creamier and may not require a layer of gloss.

Narrow Lipsticks: The most noncommittal way to wear lip color, sticks tend to create the sheerest, most natural color with only minimal defini-tion. It's the perfect thing to use in the summer or to stick in the pocket of your jeans when you go off on a bicycle for the afternoon. Lip color is not long-lasting. But it is easy enough to reapply—even without a mirror.

TO APPLY

Women sometimes ask me: "Do I really need a lip brush?" My instinct tells me that if someone poses the question, the answer is that a lip brush is probably not needed! Whether to use one or not is really quite simple: If you wear only neutral lip colors, you probably do not need to use a lip brush. A lip brush is necessary when applying more serious lip shades— red, plum, burgundy—any color that is in big contrast to your natural lip tone. Using a brush allows for a richer, more accurate application of color.

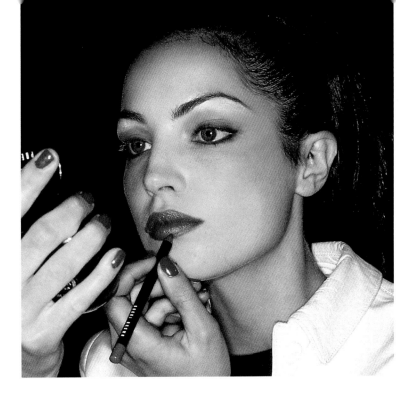

• Using a lip brush, coat on lip color. Don't attempt to paint on a shape that isn't there; follow the natural line of your mouth. Don't forget the corners of your mouth—open wide to get the best angle.

• Next, choose a lip pencil that is the same shade as your lip color (or one shade darker) to outline your mouth. Do not go beyond the natural line of the lips (i.e., don't overdraw the lip line); it looks artificial.

• Blot with a tissue, if necessary, to remove excess color and smooth the texture.

Note: For long-lasting color, use a soft lip pencil to fill in entire lip before applying lipstick.

Common Lipstick Mistakes

The Vampire Look: Pale women wearing extremely dark lipstick inevitably look like beauty victims. Even if dark lips happen to be the trend, fair women almost never look pretty in purple or nearly black lipstick; it is in too high a contrast to their skin tone. Brighter or lighter shades are more flattering. Women with darker skin, however, look amazing in dark-toned lip color.

The Brown Liner Syndrome: In the 1980s, all aspects of makeup—including lip color—went brown. One popular "brown" way to apply lipstick involved using a dark brown pencil—markedly darker than the lip color itself—to outline the lips. Some women continue to use this technique, which, I find, looks dated.

Tips: Mixing and Experimenting

What is the biggest difference between how you apply lipstick and the way I would do it for television or for a photo shoot? Most women apply one shade from the tube or tub to their mouths. I (and the vast majority of makeup artists on the planet) would be incapable of doing that. Instead, we mix together various shades and consistencies to come up with the most flattering possible choice for our subjects.

That, in essence, is what you can do if you want to be creative with your lip color and texture. Below are a few ways to pull yourself out of a lip routine so that you may have more than one look for your mouth and, in the process, have more fun with lip colors.

- Coat your lip with Vaseline and, using a lip pencil, fill in a color you like over it. This is a good way to try red or a dramatic blackberry or plum shade, since it will be quite sheer and mistake-proof.
- Put gloss on top of your ordinary lipstick. This alone will change the lip look quite dramatically. Good gloss shades include clear, white, light pink, mocha, and chocolate.

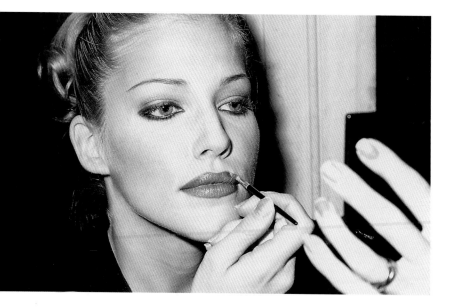

- Try using a brown-toned lipstick with a light beige lip pencil. Actually, you may use any shade you prefer—the principle being that the pencil be a shade or two lighter than the lipstick.
- Mix a chocolate lip pencil with pink shimmer lipstick or lip gloss.
- Put on one favorite lip color and then put a slightly darker shade on over it. Once you start experimenting in this way, you may find yourself incapable of wearing just one standard-issue color.

The following are some basic modulating principles that I use in my work and which may be helpful in easing into lip color that is more individual and creative.

Standard Ways to Modulate Lip Color
- White will make any lip color look pastel and lighter.
- Beige will tone down a bright shade and is a good "fixer" if you suddenly feel your lip color is too loud.
- Light pink will quiet any lip color and make it pretty.
- Blackberry/chocolate can turn a day lip color into an evening look.
- You can create your own red shade by mixing with a favorite brown.

Shape Quiz

The shape of a favorite lipstick says a lot about how you are putting it on and what, possibly, you are doing wrong.

Flat: Chances are you're applying lip color to the lower lip and then smacking your lips together to spread onto top lip. This is a good emergency measure when you have no mirror, but you risk leaving the corners of your mouth bare. (I often apply lipstick this way myself when I am in public and need to be fast.)

Pyramid: A good sign that you are probably applying lipstick individually to both lips and, if you are careful, getting the corners covered for an even look.

Drop-Off Slope: If your lipstick comes to a narrow point on one side that slopes off, you are probably placing the lipstick between the lips, pressing your mouth on the stick and running color along the length of your mouth for simultaneous two-lip application. With this technique, you risk depositing too much color at the corners of your mouth, so be sure to do a lip check in the mirror. You also may end up wasting quite a bit of the tube: In wearing it down in a lopsided fashion, the narrow part will eventually break off. It can be a messy nuisance.

Red Lips

It's been said that there is a red lipstick for every woman, and that's prob-ably true. But what good is red lipstick if you don't feel good wearing it? I personally have a hard time with red, so I always try to find ways to raise the comfort level with red.

First off, don't feel obliged to match the color red of your dress or jacket with the red of your lipstick. It's more modern not to match!

Next, don't feel constrained to wear red found in a lipstick tube—create your own customized lipstick by combining a red you like with a favorite neutral or brown lipstick.

A red lip stain is another easy way to wear red.

The lowest-voltage way to wear red? Put Vaseline on your lips, then fill in all over, using a red lip pencil.

Question: My lips are quite full. What can I do to make them look smaller?
Answer: I think full lips are incredibly beautiful. It would be my choice to put the focus on your lips, rather than trying to make your lips look smaller. Experiment with textures that you like—put a sheer gloss over a favorite lipstick. When accentuating lips, don't do a heavy eye and vice versa.

A second option is to minimize lips by wearing a neutral lip color and doing a stronger eye.

Question: My lips are always really dry. Should I be wearing lipstick, or does that further dry my lips?
Answer: When lips are dry, use lip balm that does not contain camphor, a common ingredient that is meant to be drying and healing to open sores in the mouth area. Coat lips with noncamphor balm as a base for creamy formula lipstick. Carry balm with you and reapply it as necessary. Gloss also feels great and keeps your lips soft. Avoid long-lasting lipsticks; they are drying. Eye cream is an excellent lip moisturizer at bedtime.

Question: I have really small lips. What can I do to make them look fuller?
Answer: My advice is not to try to make them look fuller. Look for medium-toned lip colors that can look pretty on a smaller mouth. You may also try lining your mouth with a lip pencil in the exact shade of your lip. Use it to the full extent of the natural mouth—not beyond the place the lip stops

and the face begins. You can also focus on your eyes instead and leave the mouth more neutral.

Question: My top lip is thinner than my bottom lip. What can I do to even them out?

Answer: You are not alone—some 90 percent of women have a thinner top lip. The best thing to do is to pencil the outside edge of your top lid only for better definition. Then apply lip color as usual. Don't try to create a thicker lip using pencil—it'll look phony.

Question: My lipstick never stays on. What can I do?

Answer: Lipstick isn't meant to stay on all day—it wouldn't be natural. But if you are looking for long wear, matte lipsticks are a good choice. Matte actually looks quite pretty as it fades away; it leaves a pretty stain on the mouth.

Another long-wear technique is to use a lip pencil in the same shade as your lipstick (or a shade lighter) applied *over* your lipstick to help keep color in place. However, avoid dark lip pencil with lightweight lipstick since, in the course of your day, you will be left with just the circle of liner, which never looks good.

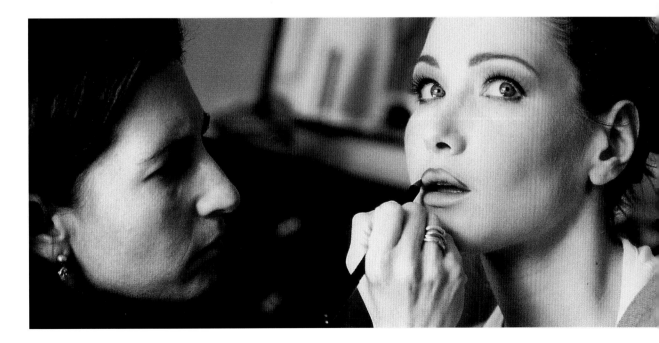

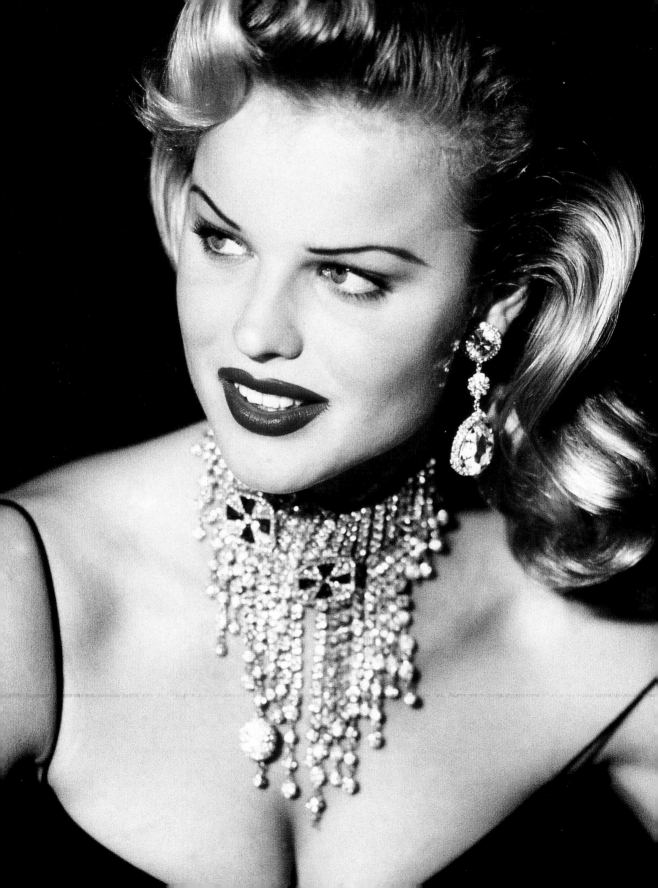

16

BEAUTY TRADE SECRETS

BEAUTY TRENDS

The makeup that appears on the runways isn't necessarily meant to be worn on the streets. Fashion shows, just like Broadway shows, are about drama and showmanship. I'm not suggesting that women ignore beauty trends, but it's a tricky balance to try to be up with the times without looking like a fashion victim. The best approach is to adapt one trend that most appeals to you and not to go to ridiculous extremes reinventing yourself every season.

If the trend is red lips (and you really love red lipstick), go for it! The toned-down version is a brown-toned lipstick that has red in it. Or find a sheer red stain or use a red lip pencil with your everyday lip color.

If the trend is black lips, the real-life option is rich matte blackberry, plum, or burgundy mixed with your favorite pink or rose lipstick.

If the runway trend is turquoise liner, try navy or gray instead.

If the trend is thick black liner, the wearable version is gray, charcoal, or slate. Or use a narrow line of the black.

If the trend is frost, put it in select spots: Use shimmer on nails, eyelids, or lips. Not everywhere.

If the trend is no makeup, be realistic. If wearing no makeup leaves you looking washed-out, do a light application instead. Keep it natural and be sure to use soft shades that warm your face and make you look pretty. Models who look like they are wearing nothing are probably wearing at least concealer, foundation, and light mascara.

If the trend is glamour makeup, save it for evening. Or wear your normal day colors, but take the extra time to line your eyes and lips. Definitely use foundation and powder—but keep it light.

DON'T TRY THIS AT HOME

Runway Beauty Practices That Don't Belong in Our Everyday Lives

Eyeliner Applied to the Inner Rim of the Eye: It only serves to make your eyes look smaller, and can cause damage to the surface of your eye.

Vaseline Applied to the Face for a High-Shine Finish: This is too greasy a look for every day. If your skin is oily, Vaseline may cause a breakout.

Bleaching or Shaving Eyebrows: Neither of these options is pretty or natural-looking; beware that shaved brows grow back slowly and, often, unevenly.

Body Makeup: A too-tanned look is old-fashioned and is almost painful to look at, given what we know about the damaging effects of the sun. Besides, body makeup can get messy once it touches garments and is difficult to apply evenly all over: Chances are, the backs of your legs won't be perfect.

Black Nail Polish, Black Lipstick: This look is too hard-edged. Opt for sheer blackberry instead.

Acid Green, Neon Orange. Look for soft, see-through versions of extreme colors, such as apricot or moss green. Or look for a quieter, more pastel take on a color you like—which looks great with bold clothing colors.

Opaque White Lipstick: Try wearing white gloss instead.

Heavy Frost: Think of it as inspiration only. A little shimmer applied on the eyelid (as highlighter) or on the mouth is a real-life pretty approach. (I never did understand shimmer on shoulders or cheeks!)

Colored or Metallic False Lashes: If you want a huge lash look, play with "conservative" black ones. Or, experiment layering three to four coats of black mascara on your own lashes.

Opaque Blue or Green Nails: This look is cute for teenagers. Otherwise, look for sheer, pretty colors.

DILUTION SOLUTION

Working the cosmetic product—layering blush, softening or intensifying shadow color, taking lip color up or down—is a makeup artist's most essential technique. Professional makeup artists often buy very inexpensive products and rely on their advanced application techniques to make these products look pretty and natural. Taking control of your makeup means developing your own layering and dilution skills. The objective is

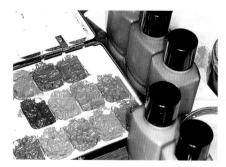

to adapt products to your liking—instead of tossing them out in frustration—thereby saving money and increasing your satisfaction.

Basic Dilution Methods

- When you use a brush with blush or eyeshadow, blow off excess color before you apply it. Blow off excess shadow and liner color from brushes, as well. If you want really sheer coverage (or are planning to layer color), use a tissue to wipe off almost all color from your brush.

- It is always a good idea to start with less color than you might eventually want. You can always layer on more color in a controlled and gradual manner. (*Removing* color from face ultimately takes more time and potentially requires going back to reapply foundation.)

- Whenever you use charcoal shadow or any other dense color, dip a brush in the product and then blow on the brush (do this over the sink or counter and out of harm's range of clothing) to remove excess. Tapping the end of a brush on a countertop also works to loosen extra color. For more intense or precise application of color, dampen your brush slightly so that shadow will adhere better.

- Clean your mascara wand with tissue to avoid a too-clumpy application.

- Dilute extreme lipstick color by mixing it with beige lipstick before applying.

- If lipstick looks too intense when first applied to one lip, use a brush or finger to spread the color thinly over both lips, thereby diluting the color and creating a beautiful stain effect. Or put a tiny bit of gloss over strong color and work over both lips.

- If you want a dewy look to the face, mix a few drops of foundation into your hand with a small amount of your daily moisturizer. If you have oily skin, mix a few drops of your oil-free foundation into oil-free moisturizer.

Corrective Measures

If you put something on your face and find it too intense, don't panic and take it off. Dilute it instead. This can be accomplished with a brush, puff, sponge, or, for the very advanced, fingers. Below, some key techniques:

- If face makeup looks too heavy, take it down with a damp sponge. Then set, using puff with face powder.

  Note: A cotton ball could also be used, but it's harder to control.

- If foundation looks too pale or too pink upon application, a yellow shade of powder will correct the imbalance.

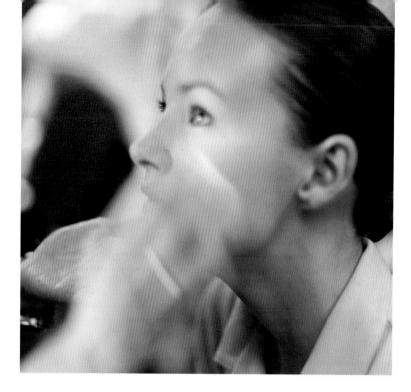

- If foundation looks artificial or masklike, rub moisturizer onto the palms of your hands or dampen your hands with water and press them gently onto your face. This will dilute your foundation. You can also mist your face with an atomizer to dilute the color. Then blend your foundation carefully with sponge or fingers and set with face powder.
- If your foundation looks uneven, smooth your face with a sponge.
- If your concealer looks cakey, smooth it over with damp fingertips.
- Too-strong powder can be brushed away with a fluffy powder brush.

    Remember: Once your skin's natural oils come through, what now appears to be too heavy may well be the perfect amount.

- If your shadow or blush looks too intense, dilute it by pressing a velour puff into some face powder and then onto your face. Or brush a clean, fluffy brush over your face to lift off the extra color.
- Soften too-bright blush by layering a neutral blush color on top.
- If your eyebrow color looks too harsh or high-contrast, press a velour puff containing a little face powder onto your brow to tone down.
- For too-harsh eyeliner, use a Q-tip or your fingertip to soften and smudge the line. If your liner is truly dense, dip a Q-tip in water or a nonoily remover to lift off makeup.

    Note: Use a non-oily makeup remover. An oily remover makes reapplication of makeup impossible.

- Blend shadow that is too dense with your finger or a fluffy brush. Or lift off the excess shadow with a Q-tip.
- If your lip color is too thick or heavy-looking, lighten it by blotting with a tissue.
- For lipstick that is too matte, blot it off with a tissue or remove it with a Q-tip. Then apply lip balm on top of what's left to create a really beautiful lip stain.
- If your lip color looks too dark, bring it down in intensity by applying beige or pale pink on top.
- If your lip color is too pale, intensify it with eggplant or blackberry lip color. These same shades can transform a day lip color into evening.
- Dilute too harsh lip pencil by applying lip balm over it.

TRICKS OF THE TRADE

I. Double-Duty Makeup

You are on the run. You have to pull yourself together quickly, but your makeup kit is back at home. What do you do? Scrounge into your bag and be creative with whatever you find. There are moments in life when you just go with it. A few examples:

- If you could only have one product with which to make yourself up, bronzing powder would be an ideal choice. Mix it with Vaseline to use on lips. Dust it over eyelids and on cheeks and at brow bone.
- In a pinch, you can use lipstick as blush. Moisturize face before applying, since neither face nor lipstick formula should be dry. (This won't work on oily skin.)
- Brown mascara is a handy all-in-one product. Use on lashes as well as to fill in eyebrows. It can even be used to cover gray roots in an emergency.
- Use clear nail polish to stop runs in stockings.

II. Makeup Cleanup

A clean latex makeup sponge works better than tissues or paper towels to lift spots from clothing. Use with a bit of soap and apply as soon as possible after stain occurs. (Non-oily eye makeup remover is also great for lifting makeup stains off clothes.)

Below are two makeup stain tricks I learned from the fashion shows. The aim is to cover stain and still be able to wear the outfit:

- Makeup on white apparel: Do not rub. Press a little club soda onto the spot and sprinkle salt on top. Let dry. If a hint of a spot remains, put white face powder or talc on top. Or use translucent powder—the only purpose I condone for this type of powder!

- Makeup on black apparel: Do as above. If spot remains, cover with black shadow.

III. Special Effect: How to Cover a Tattoo

Depending on the designer and the mood of her/his collection, it is sometimes necessary to cover a model's tattoo. I use the following method, which will work for anyone seeking to conceal a tattoo.

Find a thick, yellow-based medical concealer (companies like Covermark make heavy-coverage makeup used for covering scars, etc.). Ideally, you should purchase this makeup product in three different tones: The first product should be a perfect match for your skin tone; the second is one tone lighter than skin tone; and the third is two tones lighter than skin tone. You will be applying makeup from the lightest to the darkest shade.

Using a concealer brush, begin by applying the lightest color makeup over the tattoo to form a base. The trick is keeping the makeup only on the tattoo—not on skin. Both a stiff brush and a fairly thick concealer consistency help on this count. Then layer on the next darker shade and blend it in. Now, gently blend skin tone makeup over top. Then set with powder that matches skin tone, using puff.

DOING THE FASHION SHOWS: BOBBI'S BACKSTAGE DIARY

I always look forward to the week in March and October when I create the makeup looks for designers presenting their collections at the New York fashion shows. Since my background is in theatrical makeup, I enjoy doing a staged event. It's also a good time to push myself and try new things. Since I am known for making women look pretty, I invite the opportunity to do strong, overstated, or outrageous makeup as well.

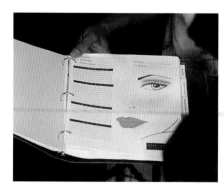

Show week is a good time get to know new models and to see my friends—designers, editors, and photographers—in the business. There are moments when it feels more like a party than work! In the end, the fashion shows are an important showcase for me.

The downside is that doing the shows is unbelievably grueling. I am on my feet for hours and, since most of the shows take place in tents, it is often hot and wet or cold and wet. One survival technique is always to have Power Bars, Emergen-C—a vitamin C concentrate—and water close at hand. I bring along a team of assistants, usually between four to eight young makeup artists, so I do have a lot of help. Nonetheless the pressure is huge. We sometimes have less than an hour to create a fresh makeup look on twelve to twenty—or more—models. Many of the models with whom I have relationships wait for me to do their makeup. So I end up supervising all the faces and doing a good number of them myself. Quite often the models arrive directly from a previous show, so we spend time taking off that makeup look before we concentrate on creating our own.

I start talking to the designers weeks before their shows. They tell me about their collections. I usually visit each designer's showroom to see the fabrics and colors (it's sometimes surprising how close to the show date the actual clothes are made up). Then I start forming ideas in my head about what I want to do. Sometimes the idea comes from a phrase the designer used, such as "country club" or "opulent" or an important color in the line. Sometimes I hear a buzzword that travels back from the European shows or from an editor I respect. I return to review my idea with the designer, often doing the actual makeup on a design assistant in the showroom. I do a different look for each designer. Sometimes, though, there is an overriding theme, like darker eyes or a richer mouth.

In the case of Joan Vass, there isn't much formal preparation. Every season she instructs me to "just do what you do." Then she'll add, "I don't want blush." Nonetheless, since the lights are so bright on the runway, I always do a little blush so the models don't look washed-out.

DESIGNERS ON RUNWAY MAKEUP ARTIST BOBBI BROWN

Michael Kors:

My clothes are not about fashion fireworks—they are about a woman, making a woman look and feel her best. The same is true about Bobbi's makeup. The most important thing to her is making the models look pretty. She is not driven by lavender eye shadow one season and then something completely contrary the next. It's never about totally veering off. We have worked together for my runway presentation for six years now. And it's never like, "My gosh! That's the most interesting makeup!" That's not the point—pretty is.

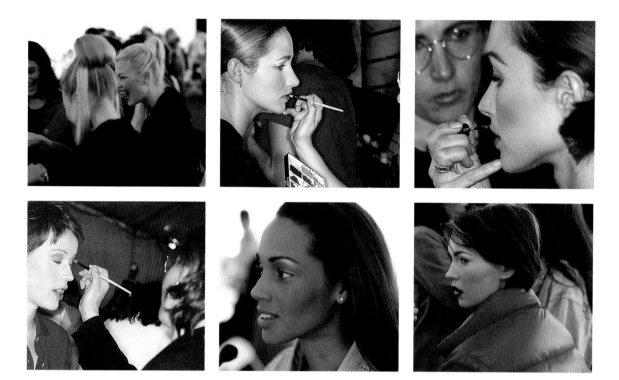

Joan Vass:

Bobbi collaborates with me so that her makeup is perfectly consonant with my clothes. She never comes in and says, "This is what I'm doing." I show her the collection and we talk things over. Then I say go for it—because I know she will look at each model and contrive to make her happy. When the models are happy, it's going to be a good show. I wouldn't call it conservative, but it isn't flashy-dashy, either. I like makeup that doesn't wear the woman.

Adrienne Vittadini:

I always love a healthy, sun-kissed look—models with a modern glow. Yes, I love glamour and things on the edge, but in the end, a beautiful look always overrules. Our vision of beauty is similar. We both love the outdoorsy kind of beauty. Bobbi gets into my head immediately. She has a wonderful karma—Bobbi must have been a Buddhist monk in a previous life. She has a very serene interior (a miracle backstage at a fashion show!). She works at a controlled pace and generates a lot of positiveness.

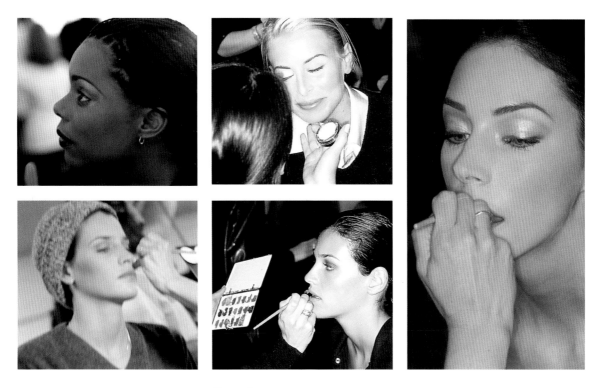

Byron Lars:

Bobbi adjusts the makeup for every model—she makes each of them look beautiful. The models always feel fabulous about how they look and that shows in how they perform. You can tell when they look at themselves in the mirror and there is that final gaze of approval. One recent theme of my show this season is Barbie—and Bobbi is perfect for this because she knows how to strike the delicate balance between trendy and pretty. Bobbi has the ability to make Barbie look powerful and modern.

Vera Wang:

For my bridal runway shows, I like the focus to be on the eyes. I love it when the cheek and the face disappear and the eyes stand out. That's very sensual and mysterious. Still, makeup is fresh with not a lot of color. This modern approach to bridal beauty is something that Bobbi under-stands instinctually and executes beautifully. The amazing thing about her is that she has so much technical knowledge but doesn't bring all the dramatics along with her. With Bobbi, there's no Sturm und Drang.

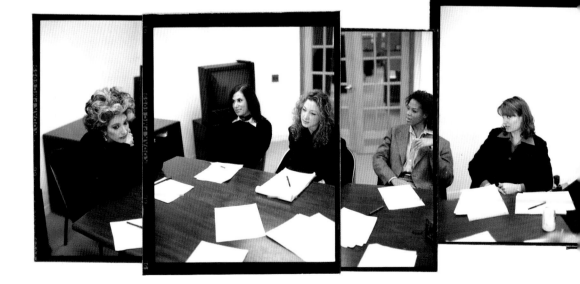

17

THE MOST-ASKED BEAUTY QUESTIONS

1. I have always worn fuchsia and pink on my lips. What's a good way to ease my way into more natural colors?

Forget switching into pale or brown lipsticks—it's too drastic a change, and you may feel drab initially. Instead, try wearing a brown-toned pink or rosy pink for a more natural look. And remember to keep using your blush to give your face a lift. (See chapter 14.)

2. How can I make my foundation look more natural?

The goal with foundation is not to wear too much, which means not needing to wear too much, i.e., having good skin. Follow a proper skin-care routine religiously. Get sufficient sleep, eat healthy foods, and drink large

Beauty Summit (below): I asked a group of friends—and friends of friends of friends—to sit down and chat with me about their beauty frustrations, confusions, and limitations. It was a no-holds-barred, honest exchange—we got so into it that, at the end, no one wanted to leave! Many of the questions in this chapter are a result of this makeup therapy session.

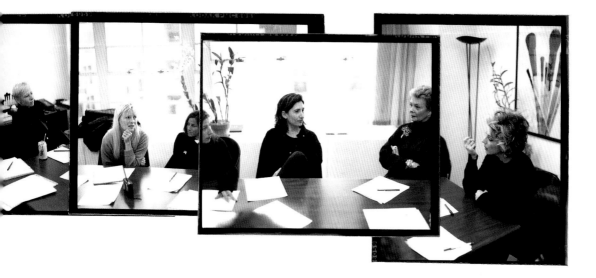

amounts of water. All of these good habits will result in a prettier complexion. In addition, be sure to buy a foundation that is the perfect color for your face. That is the single most important facet of makeup. (See chapter 11.)

3. What is a fast and easy way to change my makeup at the office to go out to dinner in the evening?

The logic behind adjusting makeup from day to night is this: Light is usually much lower in the evening, so makeup must be better defined to show up. Think about switching to a darker, deeper, or brighter lip color, such as red or burgundy. Or, if you prefer, do a pale, shimmer lip and a dark eyeliner.

4. Is there an age after which it's silly to try the beauty trends?

It's never too late to adjust your look for a particular beauty trend. If pale lips are in, for example, don't go so pale that it's not pretty. Rather, choose a flattering color that is paler than your usual lipstick.

It is completely appropriate for young girls—in their late teens and early twenties—to experiment with the latest trends. After thirty, however, each of us hopefully has developed her own beauty style and is no longer looking to transform herself with each season's newest look.

5. What's the best way to make your lipstick last?

For long-lasting wear, it is important to create an adhering surface on which to apply lip color. This is achieved by first filling in the entire lip using a soft lip pencil (you may also choose to wear lip pencil over lipstick, depending on the look you prefer). Then apply a matte-formula lipstick on top for longest wear. (See chapter 15.)

6. What are the most important areas to make up for someone who does not like to wear makeup?

Definitely use concealer to cover black circles or dark inner corner of eyes. Then, for a perfect low-commitment makeup routine, try wearing a natural blush, sheer lip color, and brown mascara.

7. What can I do about my large pores? Is there a way to make them smaller? Is there a way to make them *look* smaller?

Pore size is inherited, thus, unfortunately, there is little to do to make pores look smaller. Keeping your skin clear and smooth is the best way to assure that large pores are not noticeable. It will also guarantee that foundation will go on evenly, minimizing the appearance of large pores.

You will probably want to use an oil-free moisturizer as well as an oil-free foundation. Or you may want to try using a mattifying moisturizer that smoothes over and fills in large pores. A yellow-tinted powder will tone down any redness in your face. Be careful not to aggravate your skin with harsh scrubs or masks.

8. How do you know when to use pressed powder rather than loose powder?

Pressed and loose powder are exactly the same product; pressed powder is loose powder that has been compressed into a compact. Loose powder is more economical and allows for more complete coverage because it is fluffier; it adheres more easily onto a brush or puff.

Use loose powder whenever you are at home. Use pressed powder for touch-ups during the day and whenever you travel, since loose powder is too messy to carry with you. (See chapter 11.)

9. How can I be sure that foundation won't clog pores or suffocate my skin?

With proper cleansing nightly, your skin will "breathe" sufficiently. If your foundation feels heavy on your face, switch to a lighter formula or an oil-free version. And read the label to be sure that your foundation does not contain mineral oil. Note: If you have dry skin, you may benefit from a foundation containing oil.

10. I have always been afraid to use eye shadow. Is there an easy way to wear it so that it will look natural?

Try to find eye shadows in colors that are naturally present in your eyelid. Nothing will look more natural than that. Generally speaking, softer and lighter colors are easier to wear. Save darker shades (navy, chocolate) for eyeliner. (See chapter 13.)

11. Are bronzing powders for everyone? I am very pale, and I find them hard to wear.

If you wear the lightest shade of foundation available (say, ivory), you probably should pass on bronzing powders. No matter how light bronzing powders look, they will probably appear too orange on your skin.

Instead, play up your paleness with blush shades in soft pink and apricot. (See chapter 14.)

12. How do you prevent lipstick from bleeding while wearing gloss? I am only twenty-six, so I don't really have lip lines.

The idea is to create a matte surface on which your gloss can adhere— that way it will not travel off your lips. There are two ways to accomplish this. First, you can first apply a matte lipstick on your lips (if you want a natural look, find a lipstick that matches the exact color of your lip) and then layer gloss on top. Or, second, use a soft lip pencil to fill in the entire lip (again, choose a natural shade) before applying gloss.

13. What is the trick to blending foundation into the neck area so it looks natural?

If you must blend your foundation to avoid a visible break between your face and neck, you are wearing the wrong color foundation. The right foundation color should disappear when you apply it to your cheek. Nothing about makeup is more critical than this! (See chapter 11.)

14. I tend to get oily during the day. Should I be reapplying powder all day long? Or should I be using blotting papers or a different moisturizer?

If touching up with powder isn't enough, take a step back and consider your entire routine. Is your cleanser oil-free? Is your moisturizer? Foundation? Are you applying powder with a puff so that it will really stick in place? If skin is oily, consider skipping moisturizer in the morning and using an oil-control liquid instead.

15. I like the less-is-more concept of beauty. How can I achieve a forward, trendy look without wearing a ton of makeup?

Keep your makeup minimal and the colors muted. That way you may choose to try playing with a trend you particularly like without its being completely out of character. Do a hint of shimmer on the eye, say, or try a red lipstick that suits your coloring or a smoky eyeliner—whatever the trend of the moment. Never try more than one trend at a time.

16. How can I get a dewy, fresh look to my face without looking too shiny?

Use a richer moisturizer and skip face powder. Or use a creamy foundation formula that is not oil-free. (Note: If your skin is oily, this is not going to look good—you'll end up looking greasy.)

17. I love the way models get a bright glow to their cheeks in fashion shows. How can I obtain this look?

Take note of the color of your cheeks when you exercise—that is the shade your base blush color should be. Apply to the apples of your cheeks, and if you like a more defined, contrasted look, layer a slightly brighter blush shade on top. If you wear tawny as your base blush, soft pink would work well as your "pop" of color. (See chapter 14.)

18. How can I prevent specks of shadow from falling onto the under-eye area of my face?

It is important to blow or tap off excess shadow from your brush before you apply the shadow to your lid. Or dampen your brush slightly so the powder will better adhere. (See chapter 13.)

19. I have never plucked my eyebrows and, frankly, I have a fear of doing it. Does shaping your brows really make a big difference in the way you look?

Yes—it only takes a little brow maintenance to open up your eye. Cleaning up a few stray hairs makes a huge difference. (See chapter 12.)

20. Is there a way of making my eyelids look even and smooth without wearing a lot of shadow or putting on foundation (which tends to cake)?

Don't put foundation on your lid. Instead, use a velour puff to press face powder onto your lids. Using a fluffy, medium-sized brush, follow this with a pale, matte shadow, applied generously. (See chapter 13.)

21. I have dark hair and very fair skin. It seems like I have to use tons of eyeliner and mascara to make my eyes show up. Is there any other way to make my eyes look bigger?

Lining your eyes is the best way to make them look bigger, but you don't need to use black or charcoal. Try a softer shade of brown or gray. Then apply black mascara, layering thin coats for fullness, and bone or white shadow at brow bone to further open up eye area (see chapter 13). Also, be sure that brow is well shaped (see chapter 12).

22. I have been told to wear cool lip colors with cool blush and cool shadow colors. Does it matter if I mix cool with warm tones? Is it always obvious whether a color is cool or warm?

There are some basic rules regarding cool and warm tones. Most important, foundation and powder should always be warm-toned. In addition, blush and lip colors should both be of the same tonal family. It's up to you whether blush and lipstick are warm or cool shades; just be sure that they go together. For the eyes, the choice is whether you want shades to be warm (more natural, for day) or cool (more high-contrast and dramatic, for night).

23. What's the best way to cover up sun damage?

Use a warm-toned foundation in a rich formula. Cream blush is also recommended. Generally, it is smart to wear sunblock whenever you are going outside and to moisturize skin carefully to prevent a leathery texture.

24. How do you determine the best shape for your eyebrow?

I believe that every woman is born with her perfect basic eyebrow shape. All each of us needs to do is clean up any stray hairs (between the eyebrows is mandatory) and maintain the brow's arch at the correct place. (See chapter 12.)

25. What do you recommend for broken capillaries?

Dermatologists can "zap" the visible veins, using an electrode needle, and make capillaries disappear. This procedure can be fairly painful, so inquire first whether the doctor uses local anesthesia.

To cover broken veins with makeup, apply foundation to the area, using a concealer brush, and set with powder, using a cotton puff. If you are prone to broken capillaries, avoid extreme hot (i.e., saunas and steamrooms) and extreme cold. Excessive drinking of alcohol can lead to broken capillaries as well.

26. Even though I use powder after my foundation, I have an oily t-zone five minutes later. What should I do?

Try applying your moisturizer only on the non-t-zone areas of your face, i.e., on the sides of your face, not on your nose, chin, or forehead. Also, make sure you are using an oil-free foundation. If the problem is severe, purchase an oil-free powder and try using an oil-control lotion before applying makeup.

27. How can I keep eye shadow from "clogging" in the crease of my eye?

The best approach is to layer powder on your lid (applied with velour puff) with generous applications of nonshimmery pale eye shadow all over the lid area. Avoid applying foundation, creams, or lotions to lid. Also, avoid-cream-powder eye bases—they do not solve this problem.

28. I have allergies and a bad problem with puffiness under my eyes. What can I do?

This is a case where less makeup is more. Do not line the underside of your eye. Do not apply too light concealer (it will only accentuate the area). Keep application light and fresh. Blush on the cheeks is a good diversionary tactic.

29. How can I repeat at home what I've learned at the cosmetic counter? I never seem to be able to re-create the look.

Instead of trying to re-create an entire face of makeup, focus on picking up one or two tricks each time you go to a cosmetics counter. It may require a few trips, but, in the end, you will have a look that is totally yours.

30. Should I apply concealer under or over my foundation?

I choose to do concealer first because sometimes that is all you will need. It is important not to apply foundation over concealer, since foundation is darker than concealer and will cancel out the concealer's brightening effects. Concealer needs to be one shade lighter than your face and your foundation shade. (See chapter 11.)

31. Is there a skin cream that can reduce redness and irritation on my face?

Look for a moisturizer that is extra gentle. And under no circumstances should you use coarse grainy scrubs, Retin-A, or lotions containing alpha hydroxy acids.

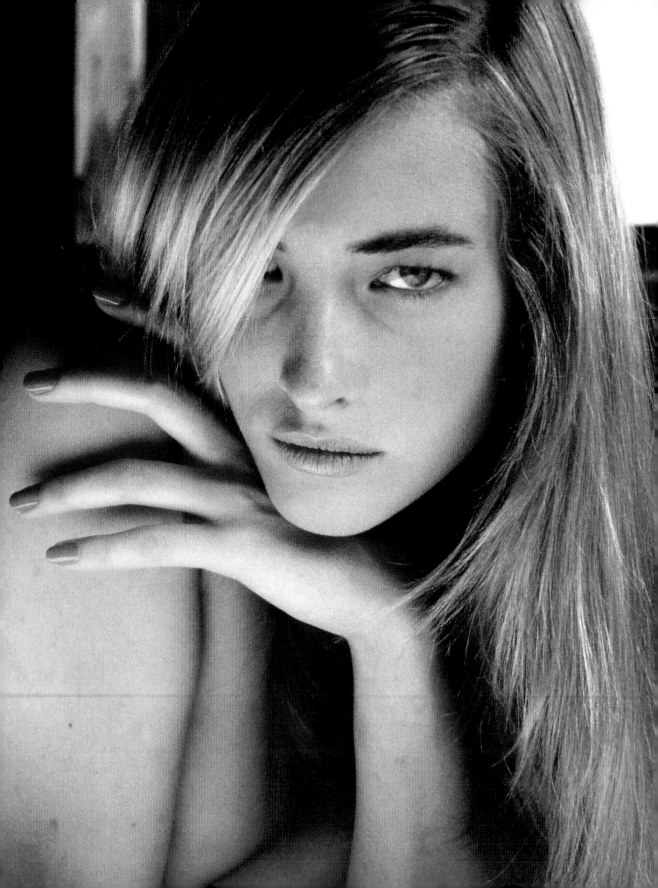

18

HOW TO MAKE IT LAST

These are among the biggest complaints: "My makeup is gone before I get to the office." "I don't have time to reapply it five times a day." "I put on twenty products in the morning, and by lunch there's nothing there."

If you are frustrated with makeup that seems to vanish, you are not alone. Lots of women face this same problem. To begin to understand what's happening on your face, ask yourself the following: Is my makeup smearing off? Or is it disappearing into thin air?

If it's clear that smearing is the problem, you should consider the emolliency (i.e., how rich, how creamy, how oily) of each of your products. There is a chance that your moisturizer is too heavy, i.e., oily—you may want to try a lighter formula or an oil-free type of lotion. Or your foundation may be too heavy, in which case you should try an oil-free one. In addition, you should check that you are locking in foundation and concealer with sufficient powder.

If, on the other hand, your makeup is disappearing into thin air (I think it must be going to the same place where all the missing socks go!), you are probably not using enough makeup or are being too subtle in your application. Think about applying makeup so that it is denser, not heavier. (This is what I'd call using a slightly heavier hand with makeup.) It may seem more dramatic than you are accustomed to first thing in the morning, but it will last.

The whole trick in getting makeup to adhere and last for hours comes down to the layering of creamy (oily or wet) and dry textures. Concealer, a wet substance, for example, will stay put only if you lock it in place with powder, a dry one. Your skin type is part of the equation, too. So when your skin is oilier, you will have to adjust with a less oily foundation, less oily moisturizer, and—most likely—more powder. I can't emphasize enough how important powder is in locking in makeup (see chapter 11). Without it, makeup is sure to evaporate.

MOISTURIZER AND LONG-WEAR MAKEUP

The key step to ensuring that makeup will really last is wearing the right moisturizer for your skin type.

Oily Skin: The big danger with oily skin is that makeup will smear off if the moisturizer underneath is too emollient. If that is your concern, check that you have oil-free formulas for your moisturizer, concealer, and foundation. If you have severely oily skin, use an oil-free powder, such as one made from corn flour.

For the best makeup adherence, use powder formulations of blush and shadows. Steer clear of cream blush and cream shadows; their creamy textures will cause them to travel. Press face powder onto lids as a base for longer-lasting shadow.

If mascara smears, it's probably because your moisturizer is too greasy. If concealer glides out of place, it is a case of too emollient a moisturizer and/or too little face powder to set it. Many women wear concealer without powder to set it, and the oil from the concealer can cause mascara to run. Powder, powder, powder!

You may find that your oily skin turns foundation a slight orange or yellow tone. To correct, try using a paler shade of powder (pale yellow powder always does the trick) over your foundation.

Even if you want every product to be oil-free, concealer looks better if it has a creamy consistency. If you tend to have blemishes, consider having a creamy concealer (to match face tone) around just to cover up spots. Look for an oil-free foundation that provides enough coverage to even out skin tone.

Normal-to-Dry Skin: Even with normal-to-dry skin, a moisturizer's emolliency helps determine the endurance potential of your makeup. In the summer, when skin is more oily, you may find that makeup is sliding off your face. In this case, you will want to wear a lighter (i.e., less creamy, more absorbing) moisturizer. In the winter months, or when your skin is dry, wear an extra-emollient moisturizer so makeup looks smooth.

Examine how you are using moisturizer—it could be that you are applying too much or too little. Adjust the quantity based on your skin's needs that day.

MAKEUP LOCK-UP: PROFESSIONAL TECHNIQUES FOR LONGER-WEARING MAKEUP

Concealer: Apply yellow-toned powder concealer with a puff to lock in place. Pile on what seems to be a ridiculous amount, then simply brush away the excess. (It's nearly impossible to put on too much powder over concealer.) As long as the powder is silky and the concealer feels and looks smooth, you will not experience "creasing" or "caking."

Foundation: Lock in foundation by pressing powder onto face using a powder puff.

Brow: While fading brow color might not be your first makeup complaint, it does reduce the strength and character of your face. There are several simple techniques to assure longer-lasting brow color.

- Use a slightly heavier hand in applying brown-toned shadow filler.
- Wet the brush before filling in brow with brown-toned shadow color. Be careful to use a light hand or it will look painted in.
- Use an eyebrow pencil (make sure it is a creamy formula for the most natural look), then dust normal brown-toned brow filler over it to set.

Liner: Use pencil liner to line eyes, then brush powder shadow of the same color on top. Or wet the brush and apply liner shadow damp.

Mascara: Use a water-resistant formula and coat on two to three thin coats, allowing each to dry a moment before moving on to the next. Thick coats clump. Save waterproof mascara for extra humid days or for special events, as it can dry lashes.

Shadow: The best way to get your eye shadow to last all day is to prime your eyelid. I take the velour puff and dust a little face powder directly onto the lid. In this way, I cover any oil while creating a smooth, dry surface on which to apply color.

In general, matte shadows last longer than creamy or frosted ones.

Blush: There are two options for longer-lasting blush, both of which involve layering techniques.

- After applying foundation but before applying powder, pat cream-formula blush on the apples of your cheeks. (Choose a really natural color for the cream blush.) Lock the blush in place with face powder. Then dust on slightly brighter powder blush.

- Layer two powder blushes—the first, a natural shade or an all-over-bronzing powder and the second, a brighter pop of color.

Lipstick: Apply an extra-thick coat of lipstick and use a lip pencil. Or use a soft pencil to fill in the whole lip and then put a stain on top. The trick to longer-wearing lip color is to alternate a dry layer (i.e., pencil) with a creamy one (i.e., lipstick or stain). Blot between coats.

Note: Do not mix powder with lipstick; the result is lumpy and gummy.

Nail Polish: Use natural shades so that chipping doesn't show. Apply a clear top coat every other day to protect color. Give yourself a manicure (or go for a professional one) twice monthly.

Fragrance: Don't try to achieve a long-lasting scent by dousing yourself with perfume. Overapplying scent will only overpower those around you. Instead, try layering a scented body cream with a light spray version of the same fragrance (eau de toilette or eau de parfum). Two light formulas will lock a scent in place in a much more pleasing way than a heavily applied perfume.

MAKEUP SELF-DESTRUCTION

Keep Your Hands Off Your Face: Without even realizing it, you may be wiping away makeup with your own hands. Catch yourself if you pull at your eyelashes, tug on your cheek, or rub your chin. Habits like these are difficult to change, but both your makeup and general comportment will benefit if you stop.

Watch Where You Put the Telephone: If you are in the practice of pressing the phone to one side of your head, you may be wearing away your makeup on that side of your face. If you work on the phone for extended periods of time, consider getting a headphone, which is also much better for your posture and alignment.

Avoid Atomizing Spritzers: Some makeup artists claim that the atomized water will set your makeup. I find, to the contrary, that it only helps speed the disappearance of makeup. (It does feel good, though.)

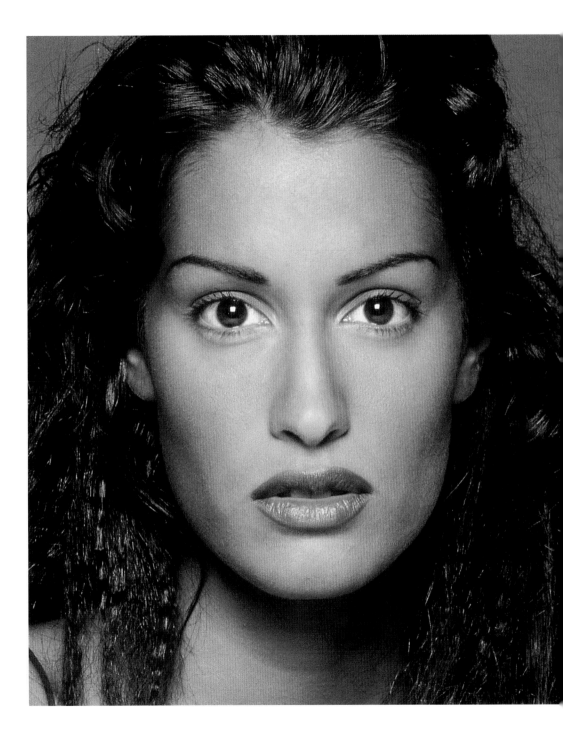

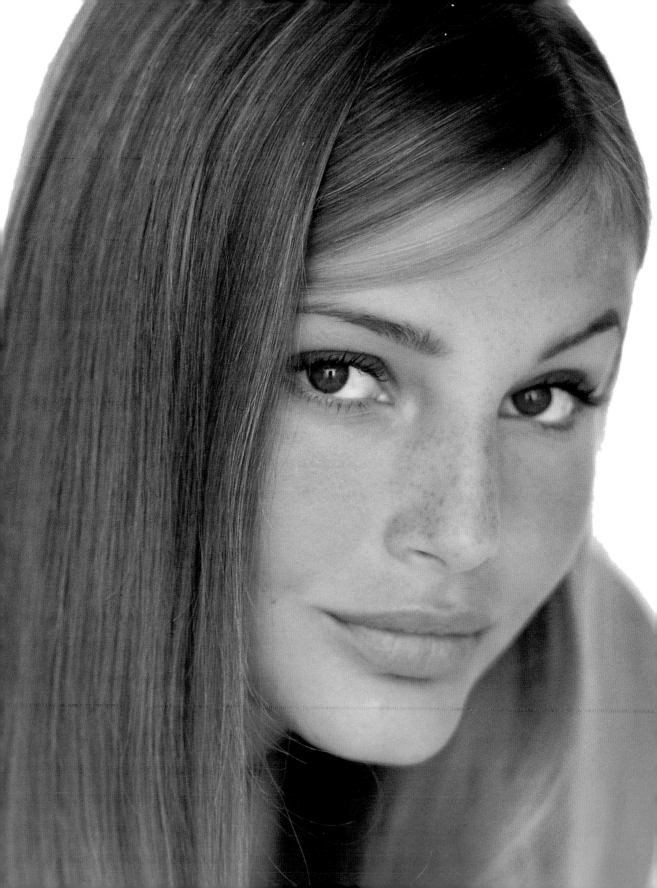

19

THE THREE-MINUTE FACE: MINIMAL MAKEUP

Three-minute makeup is the bare minimum. It's the perfect application to make you feel presentable.

Situation: It is Saturday morning and you are going out to run errands. Or you are leaving the house in the morning to drop your kids at school. You are wearing casual clothes—perhaps even sweats—and it would look wrong to do a more serious makeup. The point is not to look like you have just crawled out of bed.

1. Start with concealer under the eyes and in the most recessed corners of the eyes. It makes you look awake.
2. The next step is to deal with your skin. Put on a tinted moisturizer or, if your skin is smooth naturally, sweep a natural blush color or bronzer on your cheeks. Or, using foundation, quickly cover a blemish or redness around the nose.
3. This is a moment for brown or black mascara.
4. Wear sheer or lightly tinted gloss on lips.

Situation: You are on vacation at a beach resort. You are planning to read a book under an umbrella at the pool after breakfast at the hotel's dining room. You are wearing a swimsuit, sandals, and a cover-up.

1. Apply waterproof sunscreen to face and body before breakfast (this allows time for it to absorb and be effective). Wear sunglasses and a cap and go without foundation.
2. Wear lip balm with sun protection and lip color on top.

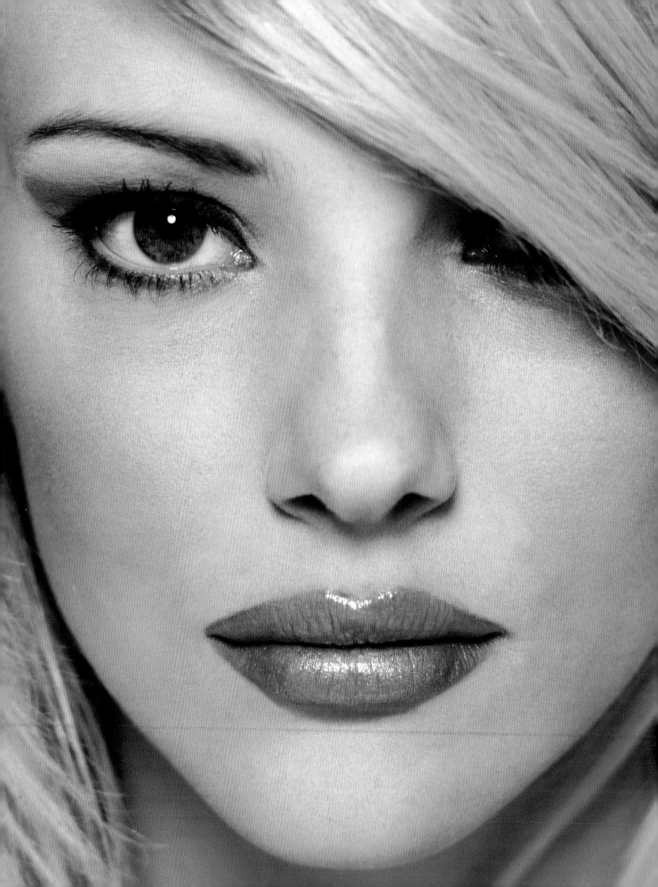

20

THE FIVE-MINUTE FACE: DAY MAKEUP

Five minutes is all you need to look pulled-together and polished. This is the makeup routine that takes you to the office, luncheons, important appointments, and daytime events. The difference between the five-minute face and the three-minute face is definition—here you take the time to define your eyes and mouth. And there's definitely more coverage with the five-minute plan.

Your total look depends on a balance between makeup and clothes. I very much like the look of very little makeup worn with a polished outfit, like a designer suit. That is very modern to my eye. The opposite doesn't work—I don't like the look of serious makeup worn with casual clothes like jeans or sweats.

1. Apply concealer first, concentrating on the most recessed corners of your inner eyes. Using the pad of your index finger, gently press the concealer to blend.
2. Apply foundation to make skin look flawless. Blend carefully.
3. Set concealer and foundation with loose powder, using a velour puff.
4. Define brow with eye shadow.
5. Use a shadow brush to dust highlighter all over the lid, from the lash line to the eyebrow. Dust medium-toned eye shadow from the lash line to just above the crease.
6. Line the eye, using darkest shadow.
7. Apply one to two coats of black or brown-black mascara.
8. Dust blush on the apples of your cheeks and blend well. Use a neutral color first, then apply brighter pop of color on top.
9. Apply lipstick.
10. Define mouth with lip liner pencil.

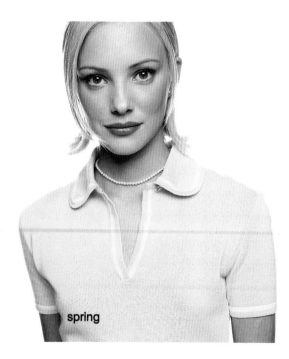

spring

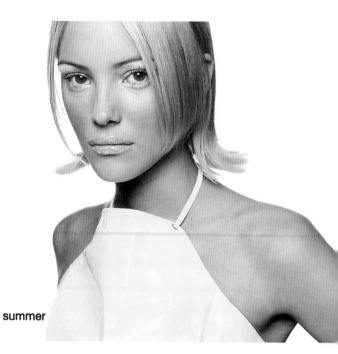

summer

21

DYNAMIC BEAUTY: CHANGING YOUR ROUTINE WITH THE SEASONS

Flexible, easy, and ever-changing—that's the essence of modern beauty style. Doing the exact same makeup, skin-care routine, or hairstyle every day regardless of the season or occasion is not only boring, but it cannot possibly be the most beneficial course of action all of the time. It is much better to take a dynamic approach to beauty. Think of change not as a burden but as an opportunity to energize, be creative, and have fun with your looks.

SEASONAL BEAUTY: ADJUSTING YOUR ROUTINE WITH THE CALENDAR

Spring is the time to:

- lighten up makeup colors: pink, beige, rosy brown, and apricot look pretty at this time of year; wear lighter textures of makeup as well
- go to a spa with your mother or a friend, or do an at-home spa day
- exfoliate from head to toe with a grainy scrub to shed your winter "layer" of skin (See salt-rub recipe, chapter 3.)

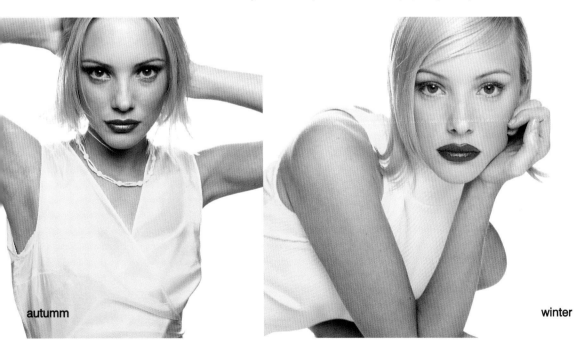

autumm

winter

- clean out your makeup bag
- get a great haircut—not on impulse, but after careful consideration
- switch to a green scent or a simple, one-note floral
- get a pedicure
- start smoothing your feet with a pumice stone in the shower
- begin an outdoor exercise routine—walking, running, rollerblading, or biking
- convert to a lighter foundation and moisturizer

Summer: For a lot of people, summer is their hands-down favorite time of the year. There's nice weather, vacations to look forward to, a slower pace, and lighter, more casual clothes to wear. Unfortunately, summer beauty is far from carefree. Heat and humidity can trigger skin-care nightmares like breakouts; rashes; tiny sweat pimples on your face, chest, and back; or extremely oily skin—as well as makeup meltdown. Air-conditioning dries your skin and lips, so, despite the heat and humidity outside, you may have to moisturize your face and wear lip balm. Balancing your face's indoor needs with its outdoor needs is tricky.

The good news is that, assuming you have a little color, you don't need as much makeup in the summer. It is a good time to simplify everything and to go as sheer as possible with all makeup products. Be conscious of keeping your beauty style as simple and low-maintenance as possible. Consider not blow-drying you hair—let it air-dry for a month.

For any prolonged time in the sun, wear SPF 30. SPF 15 is enough for everyday city wear. For a safe, tanned look, use a self-tanner (see page 166) or bronzing powder (see chapter 14).

To combat heat and humidity, switch to
- an oil-free foundation or an oil-free tinted moisturizer
- a gel cleanser instead of a creamy one
- a ponytail or easy, up, off-your-neck hairstyles
- a light eau de toilette
- talc-free body powder

Have fun with brighter lip colors and toenail polishes.

Beware of the temptation to chop off your hair on the hottest day of the year—wear a ponytail or put it up instead.

Autumn: This is a time to do "grown-up" makeup with foundation, concealer, and powder. I always think of fall as back-to-school, i.e., time to get serious. Make an appointment at a makeup counter to try new techniques or richer lip colors, such as burgundy or plum. It is also a good idea to invest in a new foundation (given the change in season and hence a change in skin tone) and to explore using bronzing powder to extend your summer color.

Now is the time to pull together your look. Clean out your closet and shop for a few key clothing and accessory items. Think about getting a new haircut.

The Holidays: This is the season to play with sparkle and shimmer in makeup. Or do a glossier mouth, say, or try a slightly reflective eye shadow.

Note: Avoid doing more than one shimmer spot on the face—do lip *or* eye—and do not put on cheeks or shoulders.

Red nails and lips are holiday staples—they always look appropriate and festive.

Devise a holiday eating strategy—think in advance how you will deal with all the extra food and drink this party season brings. Try to limit your intake at buffets and cocktail parties without denying yourself. Continue drinking lots of water and try not to break off your fitness routine.

Winter: Without a doubt, winter is the most dreary, dull time of year. Especially if you live in a region where winters are mild, the light in January, February, and March is so dull that no one looks good. Dark circles always look their darkest; puffy eyes look their puffiest. (See chapter 29.)

Makeup check:

- This is not the time of year for dark or bright colors. Instead, concentrate on warm, glowy makeup and flattering colors.
- If you tend to be paler in the winter, check that your foundation is still a proper match with your skin tone.

Body check:

- Deal with dry cuticles, a dry face, or dry hands by using richer lotions and putting oils in the bath. It is also a good time of year to do moisturizing masks.
- Put Vaseline on your nails, elbows, and heels. Buy more protective balms and ointments.

Winter is a good time of year to highlight your hair and use self-tanners. Don't fret too much if you are feeling really drab. Get good sleep, rent good movies, and just hibernate—it will be spring soon enough!

CHANGING YOUR MAKEUP WITH YOUR HAIR COLOR

Blond: Use soft pinks on lips and cheeks, and taupe and bone shadows. Blonds can also look great in salmon or peach.

Brunette: Use light-to-medium colors—rose, raisin, brown, and mahogany.

Redhead: Use rich brown or brown-red on lips; apricot or muted pink blush, brown mascara, and camel and toast shadows.

Dark Brown/Black: Deep lip colors are beautiful—chocolate, blackberry, plums, burgundies, and reds.

Gray-Hair Beauty: Does it make me look tired? Does it drag me down? These are the questions to ask yourself about gray hair. If your answers to these two questions are yes, consult a hair colorist. There are no rules about covering gray hair—and, happily, there is absolutely zero stigma surrounding it. I know women in their twenties who choose to keep their gray hair while many women start covering gray in their midtwenties.

Covering gray with the right hair shade may give you a tremendous

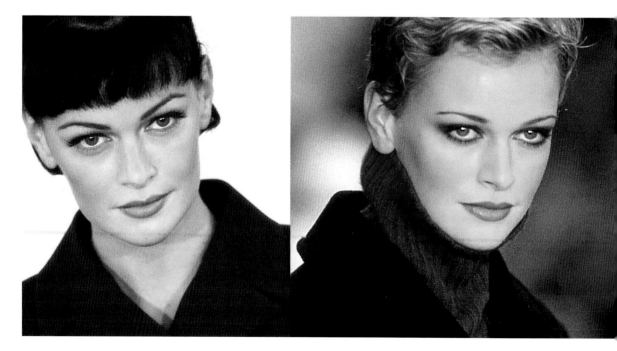

lift—you may wonder why you didn't do it sooner. Remember that hair coloring has come a long way from the narrow options of raven-black and white peroxide. There are gentle, subtle, and natural-looking options for everyone.

Tip: If you need a hair color touch-up but don't have time to get into the salon, I use a brown mascara or a color stick (Cover Gray is one that I like and is sold at beauty-supply stores) to cover the gray. Both stroke on easily and wash right out.

If you are very gray, consider asking your hairdresser to whiten your hair, which tends to be more flattering to the face. This is one way to look great with gray hair and make it your trademark.

How you wear gray hair is also extremely important: Simple shapes are much more youthful than permed and set styles. It is more modern to have gray hair and just let it fall naturally without a lot of styling fuss, thanks to a great cut. Also, I feel that the older you get, the better you look with shorter hair.

More colorful makeup is essential. Gray or white hair drains color from your face, so you need the lift of makeup color, ideally soft shades that are not too washed-out. The following are my color recommendations.

Lipstick: pink, rose, red, apricot, peach (what doesn't work: brown)
Blush: rose tones, soft brights, or pastels

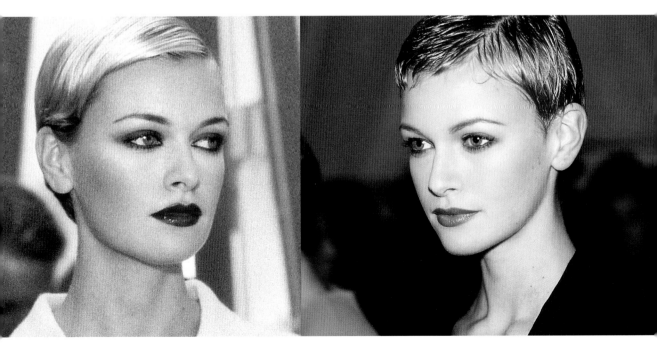

If you have brown eyes: use a gray or brown shadow palette

If you have blue eyes: use shadow trio of gray, slate, and navy

Please avoid blue eye shadow—it's very aging.

SELF-TANNERS MADE EASY

Looking healthy is my main motivation in doing makeup. Since the 1920s, looking healthy has been synonymous with having a great suntan. In recent years we've learned how dangerous the sun is for our skin; nonetheless, we still love the look of a golden tan.

Enter self-tanners. Their formulas have gotten better and easier to use every season, so they are truly a viable option. Forget self-tanning disasters of the past and give it a go—especially when your face has that unhealthy, midwinter pallor.

Some companies offer a range of self-tanner shades. If you fall between two shades, opt for the lighter one, so that any unevenness or missed spots are not obvious.

To Apply

Choose a time when you are not rushed. (I find that evenings work the best.) Exfoliate your skin first; you need to create a smooth surface. Spread on the thinnest layer of tanner possible so that any mistakes will not be glaring. If you want darker color, wait a day, then do another application.

Face: Apply the lightest coat possible. Apply around the eyes, being careful not to get product into your eyes. Do not forget your ears and neck. Your face is naturally lighter than the rest of your body, so choose a product accordingly. If you have blond or light brown brows, take care not to apply self-tanner on the eyebrows—it can stain the hairs an orange-yellow shade.

Body: Many women use self-tanners on their legs as a means to eliminate the need to wear stockings. But be subtle in application. Legs that are shades darker than arms, neck, and other exposed parts end up looking silly. Be advised that self-tanners are quite difficult to apply evenly on hard-to-reach spots like the back. In this case, look for a container with a nozzle that functions from all angles. Again, do a thin layer initially, then reapply to build color.

Note: Self-tanners are not for everyone. If you are very pale (i.e., your foundation shade is ivory) or have sensitive skin, you may be well advised to skip self-tanners all together: There may be no self-tanner light enough to look natural.

Oily or breakout-prone skin can react badly to self-tanners. If you fall into this category, try applying a thin layer on your face and leave it on for only fifteen minutes. Then wash your face thoroughly. It should be sufficient time to activate the tanning without triggering a breakout.

Warning: If possible, smell the product before buying it—some self-tanners have an unpleasant odor.

On extremely dry areas of the body (elbows, heels, knees), self-tanning lotions can leave a deep orange stain. To avoid, exfoliate these areas in the shower in the days before application. Apply self-tanner to these dry zones only sparingly.

Be sure to wash your hands thoroughly once you are finished with self-tanning application, scrubbing the areas between your fingers and the palms of your hands especially carefully. Since self-tanners can stain clothing and sheets, allow enough time for the lotion to be fully absorbed before putting on a white blouse or crawling into bed.

Question: How can I be sure I am purchasing a self-tanner that will work for me?
Problem: It's not easy. If you are very fair, it may be impossible to find a product that does not turn your skin orange. Otherwise, shop the self-tanner lines that have a choice of shade (light, medium, dark). If you are between two shades, opt for the lighter one. Feel a product's consistency to make sure that it will rub in easily.

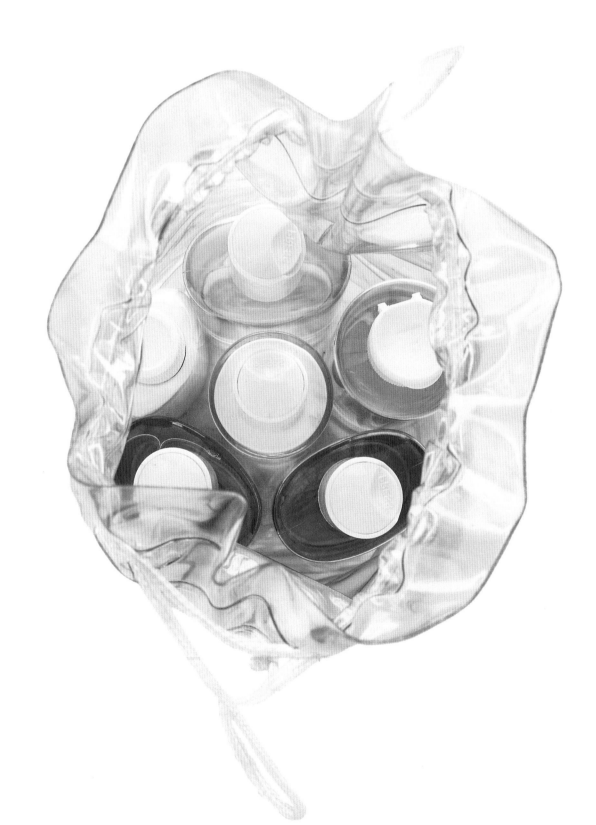

22

BEAUTY LOG: TRAVEL SKIN CARE AND MAKEUP

Travel is stressful, whether it's an overnight business trip to the coast or a dream vacation to Bali. Just getting to your destination is work; getting there looking good is even harder.

On the Plane

We all know that plane food is disgusting, but when you are stuck on a plane for hours, you somehow eat whatever is placed in front of you, sometimes out of sheer boredom. Bringing your own healthful snacks (things like fruit, dried fruits, yogurt, and whole-grain crackers or bread) as well as a bottle of water is the perfect out. Otherwise, request seafood, a fruit plate, or a vegetarian meal when booking your flight; the special meals are usually healthier and tastier.

If the trip is longer than four hours, bring face cream onboard with you. Apply a generous amount every hour or so. I don't advise drinking alcohol when flying, because it only further dehydrates your system. If you do choose to drink, compensate by drinking twice the volume of water.

Do gentle stretches in the seat: shrug your shoulders, rotate your wrists and ankles, or gently twist your upper body to one side, then the other. Get up and walk down the aisles every so often. The aim is to prevent your back and legs from becoming tight in transit. Now and then, take a few deep, calming breaths.

Beauty Jet Pack: I've learned to be organized and keep it simple: I take only the essentials. I use small portable containers and make sure that everything is nonbreakable and nonspillable. I keep a small toilet bag packed at all times. It contains things for myself and my family, and I try never to dip into these supplies so that the kit remains intact and ready to go at all times.

Basic Hygiene

- toothbrush/toothpaste in plastic containers
- shampoo/conditioner in one (small bottle)
- face cleanser
- face cream or lotion
- disposable razor (I use shampoo for shaving cream)
- children's Tylenol (for my kids)

I find that it is good to take along sample packets of skin-care products when I'm on the road. It's like taking along a lot of little treats. Sometimes I find that I have more time and energy to pamper myself in a hotel room than when I am at home with my family. This is a moment when I might do a deep-conditioning treatment for my hair or a hydrating mask for my face. I always exercise when I'm away, as it keeps me going and gives me extra energy and focus. I get up as early as needed to fit in my exercise. Sometimes I treat myself to a massage, which is almost a necessity when you travel and work. I'd rather have a massage than a new pair of shoes or a new shirt. For me, it's a priority.

Despite the hassles of travel, time changes, and what have you, I have learned to make it a satisfying experience. To wear a hotel robe, order room service, or call an old friend just to chat (and to be in charge of the remote control!) is total bliss for me.

TRAVEL MAKEUP KIT

- concealer/foundation in lip palette
- pressed powder and puff
- dark brown shadow for eyebrows and eyeliner
- 1–2 blush(es) with small-handled brush
- mascara
- bronzer
- lipstick in palette
- lip pencil
- perfume

BUSINESS TRAVEL WARDROBE (USUALLY PACKED IN A CARRY-ON)

- exercise clothes: T-shirt, leggings, Walkman, and running music
- 1 navy trouser suit (or brown, black, gray)
- 2 white T-shirts (blouses are too high-maintenance)
- socks and underwear
- family photos

I like to be comfortable on the plane, so I normally wear jeans, a big sweater, and loafers.

VACATION TRAVEL

Destination Beach: Pack your entire wardrobe of sun-protection products. Don't bother bringing foundation on this vacation—you will have your own relaxed glow. Bring blush, gloss, and lipstick. If the mood is relaxed, take a vacation from eye makeup.

Destination Ski: Pack moisturizing sunblocks and lip balms as well as rich moisturizers for your face. If your face becomes severely dry while you're skiing, apply a thin coat of lip balm instead. Beware of the "raccoon" eye–goggle tan—it looks silly once you get home. Go for pale lip colors and really minimal, relaxed makeup in the mountains.

Destination City: Bring a full complement of makeup if plans call for theater or dinner. You will probably have more than your usual five minutes to get ready, so be relaxed and pamper yourself.

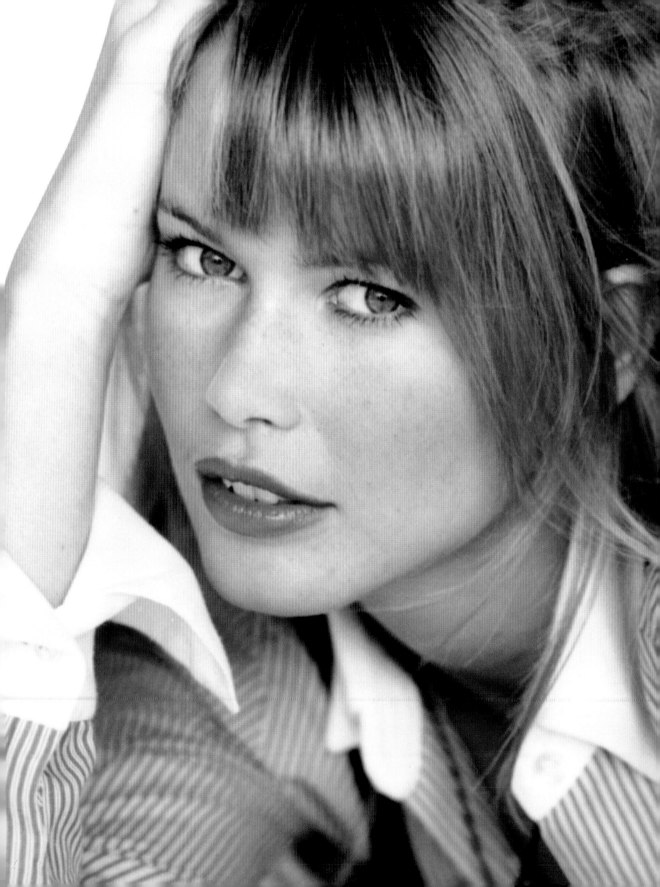

23

THE GETTING-AHEAD FACE:
INTERVIEW MAKEUP

The makeup you wear to an interview is just as important as the clothes you show up in. Both makeup and apparel send important messages to the interviewer: Is this a serious person? Is she pulled-together and professional-looking? Is she a "fit" for this business environment?

Knowing what is appropriate for a given work situation is key. Looking polished doesn't mean getting dressed up and made-up, as though you are going out dancing. Nor does it mean showing up dressed down and un-made-up, as though you are going to the gym. Whatever the job or the place of employment, the objective of interview makeup is to look pleasant and in control.

The clothes you wear to an interview can often signal the appropriate makeup. A serious, structured power suit might require a well-defined power face. This is the time for lip pencil and good eye definition via shadow and liner. Richer lip colors and eye shadows are definitely appropriate. You might even do red nails.

If, on the other hand, you wear less-structured clothes to an interview, your makeup should have less definition. Focus on smooth, clean application of your foundation rather than intense lip or eye color. Wear neutral makeup tones.

INTERVIEW TIPS

- In general, do not do a strong mouth for an interview, as it can be distracting to the person you're talking to. Use a medium-toned lipstick that is not too strong but will not need to be reapplied, either. (See chapter 18.)
- Since you will want to establish and maintain good eye contact throughout the interview, concentrate instead on eye makeup. Use neutral colors, so the contrast with your skin is not harsh. You can't go wrong with brown liner and a couple of coats of black mascara. Save more dramatic charcoal and slate liners and shimmer shadows for night.

- Makeup should look efficiently applied. The aim is to look like a serious, focused person, not like someone who spends hours in front of the mirror.
- Blush should be healthy-looking, natural, and carefully blended.
- If you are a red lipstick personality, you should definitely wear red for an interview. You might consider toning it down a bit, though. Mix your usual red with a brown-toned lipstick.
- Like the shoes you wear, fingernails tell you a lot about a person. Are they worn down or bitten? Or are they neat, clean, and short—perfectly appropriate?
- I do not like long, dark nails, nail appliqués, and nail "jewelry" in any situation—but it is especially inappropriate for an interview. If possible, get a manicure.
- Powder is key. An interview is a stressful situation—your palms and T-zone may become moist even if they are normally dry. (This is your fight-or-flight instinct taking over, but it isn't all bad. When your adrenaline is pumping, you are more up, quick, and clear-thinking.) Nonetheless, you will want to look cool and at ease. Arrange to arrive a few minutes early and ask to go to the ladies' room. Touch up with face powder and take some deep, calming breaths just before the interview.
- Your face needs to be smooth. Check it in natural light to be sure that your makeup doesn't look piled on. Use your hands to press (not wipe) excess blush and powder into your face.

Note: Fluorescent lighting can turn skin gray or pale. It can wash you out and create unattractive shadows on your face. Rose or pink blush and lipstick help counteract the unflattering, deadening effect of fluorescent light. Bronzing powder serves the same purpose. Always avoid orange and green makeup colors.

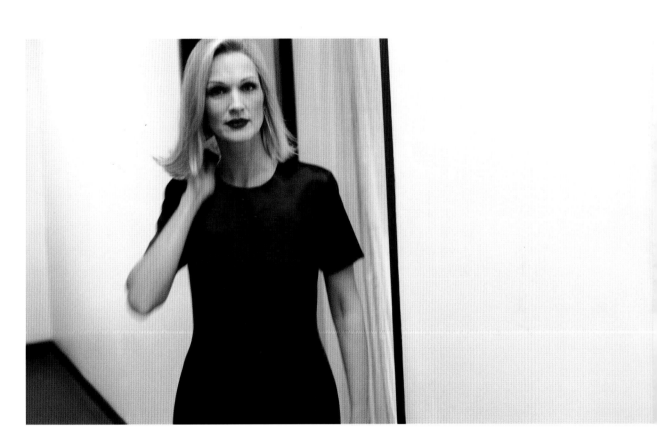

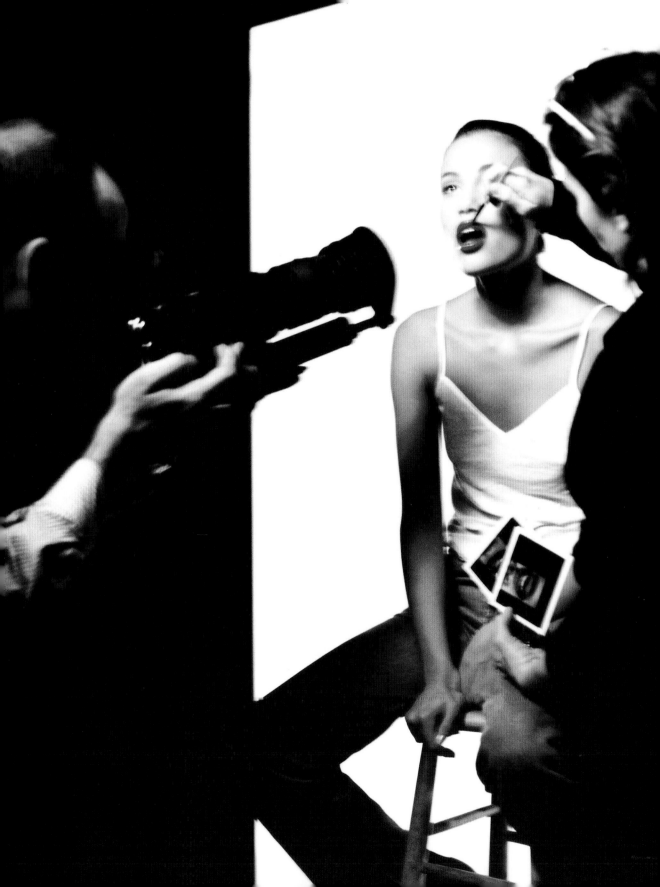

24

LOOKING PRETTY IN A PICTURE: MAKEUP FOR PHOTOGRAPHY, TELEVISION, AND VIDEO

Still Photography

Women often approach me—family snapshot in hand—anxiously demanding: "Why do I look so bad?" They are horrified at how they look in the picture and want to know what's gone wrong.

The first thing to remember is that even for the world's top models wearing the most painstaking, photogenic makeup, and shot by the world's top photographers in the most beautiful, forgiving light, it takes rolls and rolls of film—sometimes thousands of frames—to get one really good picture. The lesson for all of us is to take lots of photographs, especially if it is an important family celebration. That gives everyone time to relax. Even then, when you get your pictures back, don't judge yourself too harshly.

The right makeup, however, can help you look your best in still photography. It's best to avoid

- dark liner, since it can appear quite harsh
- too pale foundation, too pale powder
- shimmer or brightly colored shadows
- extremely glossy lips
- high-contrast colors (i.e., clashing shadow and lip colors)

How to look good in a picture: tips from two photographers. Golonka, who has taken this picture of Troy Word, who is on a set taking a picture.

Dennis Golonka: It really makes a difference if a woman gets her makeup done—or if she focuses on it herself, especially around the eyes. The other basic thing is to feel comfortable with the person taking your picture. If you don't like him or her, it will show. You won't like his or her pictures, either.

Troy Word: Forget about the camera and try to relate to the person behind it. Have a conversation, communicate. I know that sounds easy, and it's nearly impossible. I often find that when a model steps off the set to get a cup of coffee, she looks the most beautiful and real. The camera tightens everyone up—even the professionals. That also explains why some of the most flattering pictures of people are usually taken by their closest friends and family—these are the photographers who capture you at your most natural.

Flash Photography

Electric flashes have the effect of intensifying the pink of foundations and face powder in pictures, which is the reason I started using yellow-based products. Thus the tone—and undertones—of your foundation and powder are crucial. Use yellow-toned foundations and face powders. Women wrongly assume translucent powder is invisible—it's not. It can drain the color from the face and look masklike in flash prints. Translucent powder is the number-one reason women look bad in photos!

Paparazzi Pretty

It's hard to look your best in candid flash photos, but warm tones of powder and foundation help prevent the washed-out flash look.

Black-and-White Photos

Good definition is the key to makeup for black-and-white photography. That means careful lining of the lips and eyes and well-applied blush.

Warm v. "Blown-Out" Lighting

The type of makeup I do on photo sittings varies dramatically depending on the photographer's lighting. With harsh, high-contrast studio lighting, blush becomes very important to the definition of the face. Eyes and lips can be stronger in this situation. One's flaws are softened with this type of light, but skin appears cool and flat in the picture.

Conversely, with warm, golden light (often late-afternoon, diffused natural light), minimal, natural makeup is the best approach. This is the ideal working condition for me, since it's my definition of pretty: warm skin tone and a healthy golden look.

Daylight Photography

Natural lighting is very realistic. *Everything*—too much makeup and any imperfections—shows up on the film. I recommend doing minimal makeup, using enough concealer and foundation to even out spots or redness (as in around the base of the nose and around the mouth).

General Photo Tips

- Try not to be nervous; your facial muscles will tighten and you will not look like yourself.
- If your nose looks big to you in pictures, you are probably dropping your chin. Make a point of lifting your chin next time. Lifting your chin will also make dark circles appear less intense.
- If your portrait is being done, close your eyes between shots. Take a deep breath and then open your eyes. You don't want your eyes to

look too intense, so don't stare into the camera. Soften your focus instead.

•Tilt your head; move your face. Try not to act frozen.

Question: When my picture is taken, my face looks whiter than my chest and arms. How can I prevent this so I can look more natural?

Answer: It is normal that your face be lighter than other body parts due to the proper use of sunblock, and more frequent cleansing. To counter the appearance of a lighter face, use a half-shade warmer foundation or mix your regular shade with a slightly darker one. You may also want to use a warmer powder. The neck area also tends to look light, so it's a good idea to warm up that area with bronzing powder.

TV/Video Makeup

On film, everything is magnified one million times, so the fundamental makeup objective is major coverage. All makeup must be applied more heavily and more matte to counteract the harsh lights of television or video. Don't worry if it doesn't look pretty to your eye when you look in the mirror.

Foundation: Use creamy, heavier-than-usual matte foundation. Or use your regular cream or stick formula, just more of it. Television turns foundation paler and orangey, so choose a yellow-toned foundation that matches your skin tone but is one half-tone darker. This is a moment to mix your own foundation—the dark and medium shades—for the desired effect. Makeup should not look cakey and pasty.

Concealer: Use more concealer than usual—two coats at least in a shade that is slightly lighter than your normal concealer shade (i.e., mix your regular concealer with a lighter shade).

Powder: Use *lots* of it. The ideal is to have three shades on hand—your normal shade plus one shade darker and one shade lighter. Over foundation: Choose one half-shade darker face powder to warm your complexion. (Mix a one-shade darker powder with the normal shade of face powder.) Over concealer: one half-shade lighter powder generously applied to eliminate the appearance of dark circles. (Mix a one-shade lighter powder with your normal shade of face powder.)

The more matte, the better. The finish of your face should be matte, not dewy. Don't worry about the appearance of lines—the strong lights will blow them out. Even the tiniest bit of dewiness or moisture on the face will look like grease on film.

Define: Carefully define brows and eyes, but avoid extremely dark shades.

Blush and Lips: Rose, red, and pink tones look pretty on television. Color needs to be brighter than you are accustomed to wearing for day, but not Day-Glo bright.

Best to Avoid

- Orange-toned blush, lips, and foundation.
- Blush and lip colors that are too soft—you could look washed-out.
- Shimmer shades will look greasy.
- Beige or brown lip tones—you need a little bit of brightness.

SOME OF THE BEST TV MAKEUP AROUND

Oprah Winfrey: A great on-air role model, her makeup is always flawless and never exactly the same. Oprah likes to experiment with browns, plums, and charcoals.

Jane Pauley: Grays and navy bring out her blue eyes. Pink and coral on her lips are soft and pretty without looking washed-out.

Katie Couric: Bright lips are her trademark. Her makeup always comes across as fresh, natural, and pretty.

Paula Zahn: She is the epitome of outdoorsy fresh, with tawny and healthy tones that never look drab.

Joan Lunden: She wears softly bright colors and communicates fresh and pretty.

Ricki Lake: Wearing modern browns and plums, she has the most current makeup on television.

Sally Jessy Raphael: Red lips are the focal point of her simple, classic on-air style.

Diane Sawyer: Her makeup palette is always classically blond—lips are pale pink or salmon, the eye is done in taupe, sometimes with navy liner. It's clean and simple.

Candice Bergen: Sitcom anchorwoman Murphy Brown wears subtle, modern makeup: healthy outdoorsy cheeks, brown eyes, and light-to-medium lip colors.

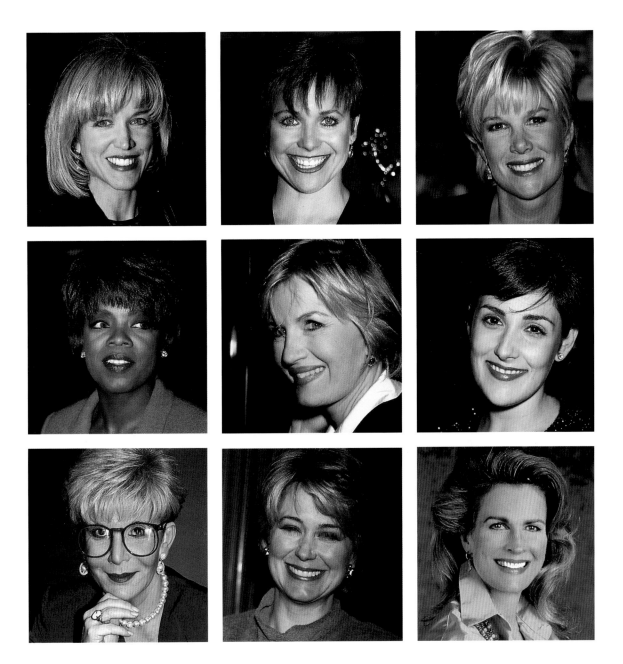

VOGUE

SEPTEMBER $4.00

THE BIGGEST FASHION ISSUE!

FALL
THE MOST EXCITING LOOKS

25

AFRICAN-AMERICAN BEAUTY

The first time I did makeup on a black model it was a disaster. It was in the early 1980s, at the beginning of my career, when I was doing a test day in a studio. (Test connotes that there is no advertising client or magazine assignment per se. It is an opportunity for young talent—makeup artist, model, hairstylist, and photographer—to experiment and, hopefully, get beautiful pictures for their books.) I worked for a long time applying the foundation on this young model's face. But when I had finished, my mistake was clear to everyone: I had made her look gray. My test day was a flop.

Determined to get it right, I started buying foundations in an effort to find the very best shades manufactured for African-American skin. After spending a lot of money and time, I discovered that there are very few good shades out there. At that moment, I began to understand black women's frustration with the cosmetics process. The marketplace was filled with foundations formulated (for the most part) by white people—oftentimes white male MBAs—for white people. Since then, the market-place has changed, thanks in part to ex-model Naomi Sims, who created a makeup line specifically for women of color. The big cosmetics compa-nies followed, adding broader shade ranges to cater to a more ethnically diverse consumer base.

Part of my education came from looking more closely at black women's skin so as to recognize the variances in undertone. I learned that some black women make up their faces to match the lighter tones of their skin, bringing "up" the darker areas. Others (and this is the approach I prefer) opt to warm the lighter tones to blend with the darker tones of the face. Of course there are black women blessed with the most flawless, even-toned skin. Most, however, have to contend with a range of different colors.

I also discovered just how ingenious and talented a lot of black women are with their makeup because they have had to be. Many learned to be their own makeup artists, mixing their own perfect foundations.

I knew I got it right when, in 1993, my first American *Vogue* cover was a photograph of black model Naomi Campbell. (It also happened to be

Naomi's first *Vogue* cover.) The picture was taken on the beach in East Hampton, Long Island, by French photographer Patrick Demarchelier. The makeup dispute this time, however, wasn't about foundation. Naomi has a trademark lip technique: She likes to line her lips dark. I decided to make her lip all one color instead. (In this case, I chose a blackberry stain.) The set was outside, and there was no mirror for her to check it out. I thought it looked beautiful, Patrick and *Vogue's* stylist, Grace Coddington, liked it. And so, evidently, did the editors at the magazine and its millions of readers. Naomi, however, couldn't be convinced.

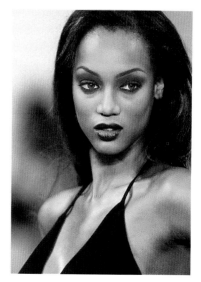

FINDING A FOUNDATION THAT WORKS FOR YOU

It's a good idea to have three different foundation shades on hand to allow for the different gradation of color on your face. This is definitely a place to learn to be your own makeup artist, blending and mixing different shades for different areas of your face. Lots of black women are darker across the brow and chin and slightly lighter on their cheeks. To even out this differential, apply a lighter foundation shade on the forehead and chin areas and a slightly darker shade on your cheeks. Blend carefully.

- Light concealer/foundation is your concealer color, which should be used under the eye, but can also be used to lighten a dark forehead or chin area.
- Medium foundation (or one shade darker than concealer) is your all-over foundation color, to be used to correct spots of varied pigmentation. If you get more color in the summer, medium will then become your concealer shade.
- Dark foundation (or one shade darker than foundation/two shades darker than concealer) is used to even out the lightest areas of your face or as all-over foundation when you have a tan.

Note: Experiment with a bronzing stick to bring down the lighter tones of your face.

Texture: Good coverage is important—look for a creamy, soft finish. Avoid any foundation that looks pasty, masklike, or cakey.

Tone: The starting point is foundation that has yellow undertones. Beyond

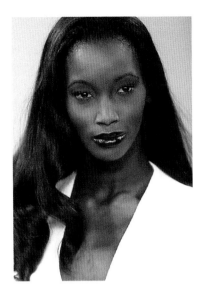

that, the right foundation depends on the depth and tone of your skin. If you have very dark skin, a foundation with a slight blue cast works best. If you have medium-toned skin, choose a foundation with a red-yellow hue. If you have light skin, look for a soft golden foundation shade. Or try mixing yellow with red or blue for a perfect match. Another option is to use bronzing stick as your foundation to warm your complexion.

OILY SKIN

Sometimes oily skin has an hard upper layer. Regular exfoliating is essential to keep skin soft and smooth.

Try using a mattifying cream (one that dries to a matte finish) before you apply foundation. If your skin is very oily, don't use a moisturizer at all during the day and use an oil-free moisturizer at night.

Oil-free foundation is a must.

Don't be afraid to use a lot of powder to seal your concealer. (This is true for everyone, but especially important for women with oily skin.) Use a brush to position a generous amount of face powder onto your concealer. Then dust away any excess powder with the brush.

The darker your skin, the shinier it appears to be. If you find that powder makes your face look ashy, skip it. The darkest skin tone often looks best with oil-free foundation and nothing else.

Note: If you have severely oily skin, you may want to try an oil-control lotion, which helps stop oil from seeping through foundation. Lots of models use oil-control liquids to keep their skin dry-looking in front of the camera and hot lights.

Blush: The key thing is to avoid any blush that looks ashy on skin. Lighter skin tones look pretty and natural in dark bronzers. Apricot, rose, plum, and soft pink also work well. Medium to dark skin tones need deep blush hues, like deep rose, currant, and plum. Dark skin tones often look best as is—skip the blush!

Question: What should I do if my bottom lip is paler than my top lip?
Answer: There are two courses of action. The first is to even out your two lip colors. Put a sheer, dark lipstick on the lower lip as a base. Then apply the same lipstick over both lips.

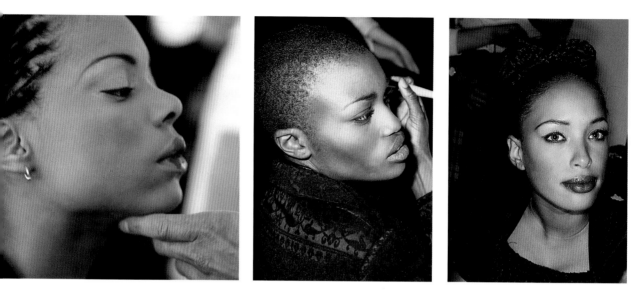

The second approach is to play up the difference. (Some people call differing lip tones a flaw; I call it a distinguishing feature!) Apply a light pink to the lower lip and use a dark chocolate lip liner.

Question: How can I minimize the size of my lips?

Answer: When I make up a black woman I often get the complaint "My lips look so full!" I feel like saying, "Well, those are your lips and they are beautiful!" I think that most black women have incredible lips, and my instinct as a makeup artist is to highlight them. It's ironic that white women run to get silicone injections to plump up their lips, and black women seek to minimize the size of theirs.

Nonetheless, if you want to downplay the size of your lips, don't line with pencil and don't wear bright, attention-getting lipsticks. Chances are you don't need a lip pencil anyhow—I find that most black women have perfectly shaped and defined lips. Wear quiet and flattering lip colors like caramel and soft brown.

Question: How do I choose lip color?

Answer: The lighter your lips' natural tone, the lighter your lipstick. If a lipstick looks pretty on your friend, don't assume it will work for you. Steer clear of ashy, pale colors. If you like pale, find richly pigmented pale lipsticks. At all costs, avoid the 1960s pale lip look of Diana Ross and the Supremes. We're over that!

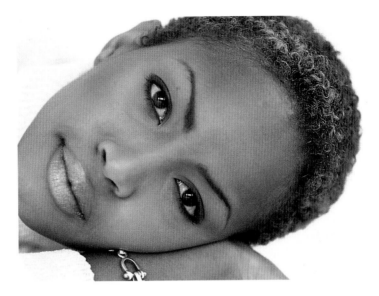

Question: How does my skin tone relate to my lip color?

Answer: In general, the darker your skin tone, the darker your lip color. Burgundy or blackberry are beautiful on dark skin. Women with medium skin tone look pretty in currant or red. Those with light skin tones look gorgeous wearing low-voltage neutrals and glosses.

Question: What's the most modern lip look for African-American women?

Answer: Deep but sheer lip color is a modern, natural look for all black women. Chocolate lips are a favorite of mine. If you usually wear brights, ease into a browner lip by mixing a deep brown with your usual bright. Deep reds and browned reds are the most flattering on dark skin, while brighter reds and orange reds stand out too much and do not comple ment most skin tones.

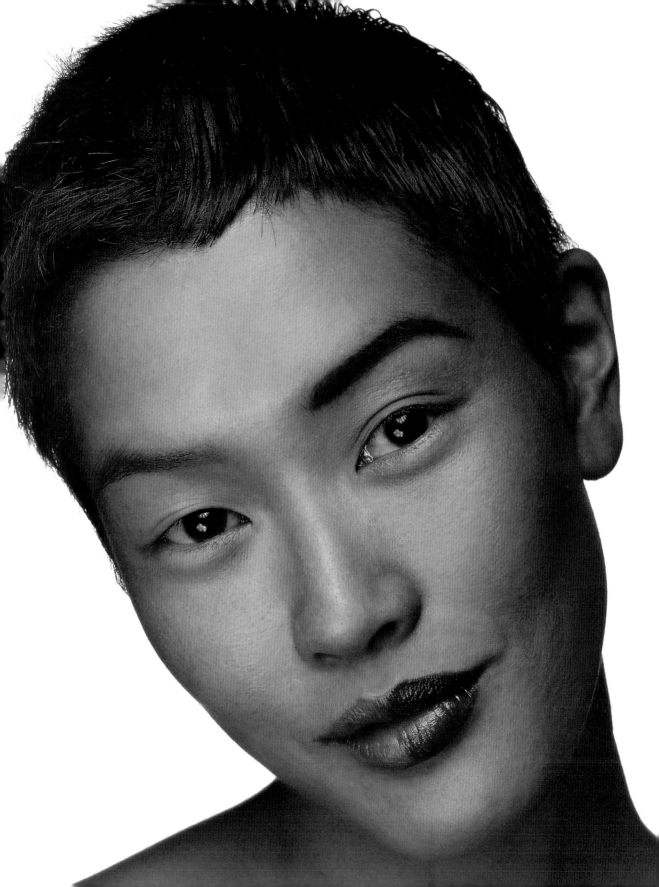

26

ASIAN BEAUTY

"How do I make my face look smaller?" "How do I make my eyes look bigger?"

These are two questions I hear all the time when I travel in the Far East and when I meet Asian-American women at home. I always register these women's concerns, but I cannot offer an easy color trick or application technique as the solution. Instead, I talk beauty philosophy. Asian beauty is characterized by round, smooth faces and thick, gorgeous hair. I urge Asian women to take stock of their many unique and beautiful features and not try to appear Caucasian. I believe that Asian women are among the most beautiful women in the world.

In general, I think Asian women look their most beautiful when not wearing a lot of makeup. I recommend a light-to-medium hand at most.

Fundamental to my approach to Asian makeup is the use of yellow-based foundation and powder. I encounter a lot of Asian women who are reluctant to try any product that is yellow-based. For years, Asian women were instructed to wear pink makeup colors to counteract their natural skin tones. But I feel adamant that pink- or red-based makeup looks old-fashioned on Asian women—it perpetuates a very unmodern "china doll" look.

Asian women fear that they will appear more yellow doing it my way. Yet I assure you that an Asian woman will not look more yellow wearing a yellow-toned foundation: She will look flawless, as though she were wearing no foundation. Nothing is prettier or softer.

FOUNDATION

Use yellow-toned tinted moisturizer or foundation. Pink-toned foundations look old-fashioned. The same is true with face powder, where you will also want to use a pale yellow shade. Even if this sounds contrary to everything you have ever thought about makeup, try it. You will be pleasantly surprised with the results.

EYES

Brush a light shadow color all over your eyelid. Then use a medium color from the lash line to three-fourths up the lid.

Liner is key to an eye look you will love. The trick is to make a thick, smoky line, not a thin, hard one. Note that the line should be thick enough so that it's still visible when your eyes are open. Apply liner all the way around the eye, with the upper lid lined in a much heavier fashion.

Fill in your brow using a hard, slanted brow brush and a brown-toned shadow. Defining the brow adds strength to the face. This is a step that is often overlooked or neglected but has the potential to enlarge the entire eye area.

MASCARA

It is ironic that so many Asian women have thick, beautiful hair and often only sparse eyelashes. If your lashes are abundant enough to wear mascara, use a thickening mascara and do three layers, allowing a minute between coats for drying. If your lashes are long enough to curl, do so.

If your lashes are extremely thin, do not try to achieve a thick-lash look. Instead, apply a smoky powder liner at the lash line in a dark brown tone. This technique has the same effect as thick lashes.

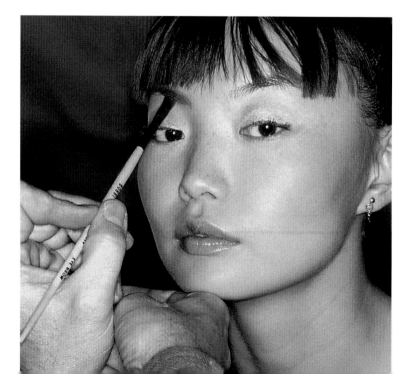

BLUSH

Apply blush high on your cheeks, toward your hairline—not on the apples of your cheeks, since this can make your face appear wider.

Choose rose or tawny shades if you have medium-to-deep skin tone; soft, pale pinks look pretty on pale skin.

LIPS

I think Asian women have the most beautiful lips; they can look amazing either in rich or extremely soft colors.

Experiment with deep-toned raisin or clove shades—rich spice tones look especially pretty if your lips are full and dark-toned naturally. In general, red-brown tones look better than orange-red ones. Or try pale lip colors, especially if your natural lip tone is light. Pinks—even the palest pinks—can be extremely pretty.

COMMON EYE MISTAKES

- Too-dark eye shadow colors that make the eye look smaller
- Contouring in an effort to create an eyelid—this is almost always a bad idea.

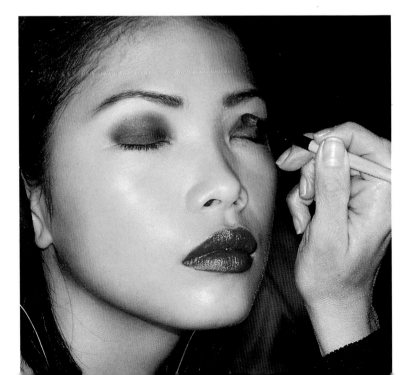

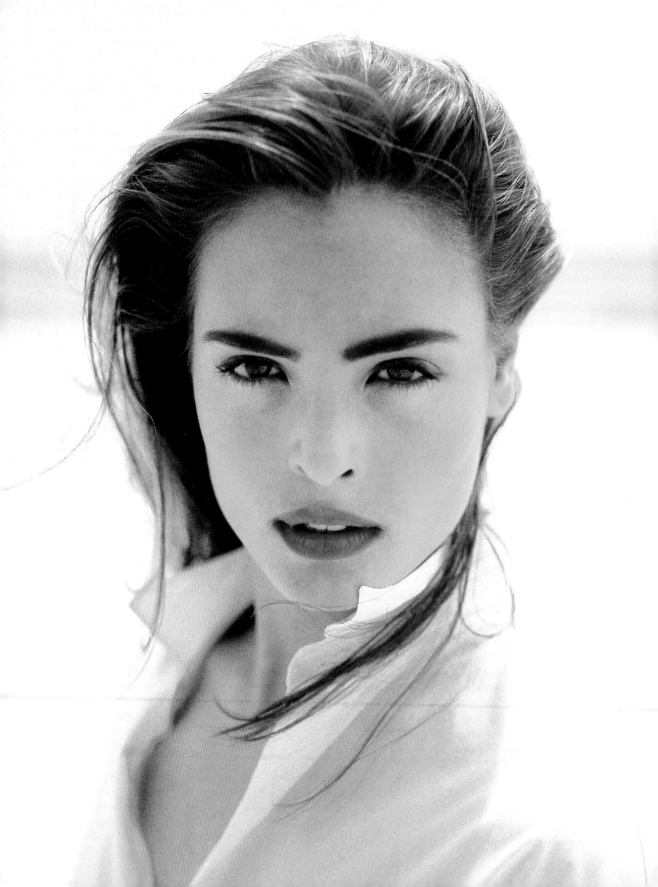

27

LATINA BEAUTY

COLOR

Think of a pop of color somewhere—not everywhere. Avoid fuchsia lips and jewel tones—they are cliché colors for Hispanic women. Think about deeper and richer—not brighter—colors, such as wines, plums, deep pinks, and rose.

LIPS

Many Hispanic women have a beautiful, dark natural color to their lips, so deep lipsticks are natural-looking and lovely. Softer tones can also look pretty. It's best to avoid brights, oranges, and loud corals.

FOUNDATION

Hispanic women most often have yellow-orange undertones to their skin. Look for yellow-orange foundations and tinted moisturizers to match your skin tone.

Question: My skin looks green in the winter. What should I do?
Answer: This is a common frustration for Hispanic women. A deep bronzing powder will give you a warm, tanned look and make you feel great (see chapter 14). Don't forget to apply a pop of color on the apples of your cheeks.

Remember that rosy colors—not orange—work best in counteracting a greenish cast to the skin.

Question: I have thick, bushy eyebrows. Should I bleach or wax them?
Answer: Shape your eyebrows by tweezing or waxing (see chapter 12). Do not bleach brows unless you lighten your hair color. Brow color should balance hair color.

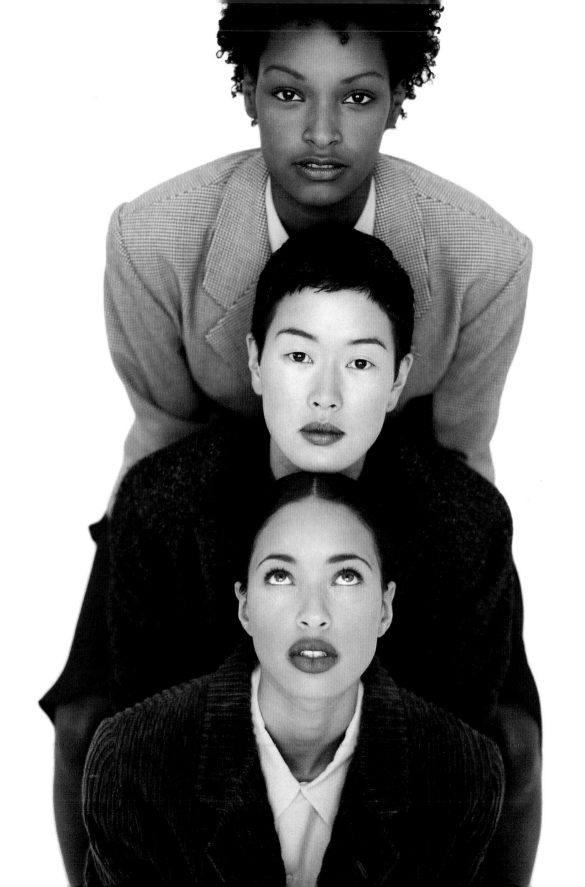

28

GLOBAL BEAUTY

Over the past decade, a whole new classification of beauty has emerged. Its hallmark is ethnic diversity. Almost by definition, global beauty implies exotic, thoroughly individual characteristics (which makes defining it nearly impossible).

What is fascinating to my eye is the exotic mix of traits. I never am able to identify what a woman is exactly—other than beautiful. I often ask models where their families came from, just to know. The answers are a testament to how very small our world has become: German, Asian, and African-American; or Irish, Native American, and Italian; or Swedish and Central African. Despite their current acclaim on the modeling circuit today, these global beauties have in the past been left out. They are not white, not black, not Hispanic, and not Asian. They are perfectly unique.

MAKEUP FOR EXOTIC SKIN TONES

Unfortunately, not many companies make foundations that look natural on exotic skin tones. The best approach is to look for golden-yellow skin colors. Remember, if the product looks ashy on your skin or if you must blend it really carefully, it's wrong.

The good news is that you probably look best with very little makeup. Foundation, powder, and blush might just be enough. Too much makeup and too bright colors will detract from your beauty.

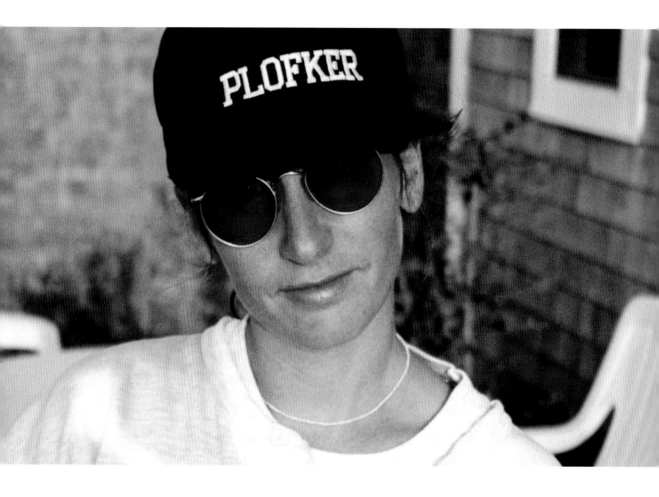

29

BAD-DAY BEAUTY

What to do on a nightmare morning—the kind of day when you look into the mirror and something has gone seriously wrong with your face. Since no one ever knows how or when a bad beauty day will hit, it's best to have a variety of solutions at your disposal, i.e., different options for different disasters.

Things That ALWAYS Make You Look Better

- The best way to turn a bad day around is to do something cardio-vascular. Go for a run, fast walk, or swim. Exercise will get rid of the puffiness in your face and open up your pores. It will help energize you for the day and will always make you feel better. Try to go for an aerobic session of twenty-three minutes (the threshold for boosting metabolism), but if you're short on time, do whatever you can. Even ten minutes will help. If possible, do your activity out-of doors.
- It is always good to concentrate on the face. Take five extra minutes to do a moisturizing mask (not a drying clay mask, but a hydrating gel or cream solution) or a scrub.
- Another big help is to put extra moisturizer on the face to soften it and plump it up. Remember to give creams and lotions a few minutes to absorb.
- Use concealer and tinted moisturizer rather than foundation on a bad beauty day. Foundation can actually accentuate tired skin and appear heavy on the face.
- Drinking water helps a lot. Try to drink a liter bottle of spring water in the morning—add lemon if that helps you drink more.

Makeup Options: Depending on the Day

Sometimes, when I'm having a really ugly day, I just want to wear lip balm and concealer. Anything more and matters would just get worse. Other times, a soft pink blush is just the thing to brighten my face. Bad days are

What do I do on a bad beauty day? I wear a baseball cap *and* sunglasses.

times when less is more. I tend not to do much with my eyes. Nor do I make a big color statement with my mouth.

If you can't be in complete control of the way your face looks, you might consider taking extra care with other elements of your appearance. The idea is to take attention away from what you don't like and put it some-where else. Wear a funky pair of shoes, a bright scarf, or a great hat.

Pearls (real or imitation) draw flattering, reflective light to the face. Wearing pearls is an age-old beauty trick made modern by Coco Chanel, who piled on real pearls with fakes, long and short strands. Both Barbara Bush and Jacqueline Onassis have made pearls a signature. A multi-strand choker also works nicely to cover neck imperfections.

Choose to wear clothes that make you feel both pretty and comfort-able. Spritz on a fresh cologne that contains "up" citrus or fresh green notes to give you a lift. Take extra care styling your hair so that it makes you feel good.

If you don't need to dress up, try wearing a baseball cap. Wear sun-glasses when you go out.

Problem: Sick-looking or extremely pale skin

Solution: Focus on skin care. Take a few extra minutes in the morning to do a soothing mask. Don't try to overcompensate for your paleness with bright colors. Use only neutral blush and shadow and lip shades to add some warmth to the skin.

Problem: One glaring pimple

Solution: The temptation to attack a pimple with your fingers is huge. But try to resist touching or popping it—that will only make matters worse.

To cover a pimple, apply foundation using a concealer brush. Press a little powder on top to set. Repeat, layering foundation and powder until blemish is well hidden.

Problem: Extreme puffiness

Solution: A heavy-lidded feeling in the morning is usually the result of too heavy food, too little sleep, or too much alcohol the night before. This is the kind of morning I try to do less, stay calm, and just go with it—accept-ing as a premise for that day that I will be tired. A cup of coffee might just make matters worse, so start off the day drinking water and setting prior-ities for the day. (Sometimes a cold compress on the eyes can help.)

The most common mistake for puffiness is to overdo your eye makeup. Do only a sweep of neutral color on the lid. If you need more definition, use a medium shadow on the lower lid instead of your normal, dark shadow liner. Whatever you do, go minimal with sheer, natural makeup.

Problem: Extremely black under-eye circles

Solution: Pay particular attention to concealer application. Do two coats of concealer, then lock it on with pale yellow powder. To help keep under-eye area open and bright, do not wear mascara on lower lashes and do not line your eyes. Choose warm, flattering, and soft colors for blush and lips: a soft pink blush, for example, and a soft brown-pink lipstick. This would be a good day to wear gloss over lipstick to reflect light and draw attention away from eyes.

Problem: How to look good when you have a cold

Solution: Moisturize! Use a yellow-toned creamy foundation around the nose to counteract the redness. Lock foundation in place with yellow-toned powder. Be careful not to use concealer that is too light. Brush on only a hint of blush in a soft pink or rose shade—but don't do too much. Keep your eyes simple.

You will probably need to touch up around your nose during the day, so carry a small amount of foundation and powder in your bag.

Problem: Sunburn

Solution: This is a time to do anything possible to soothe your skin. Wear an extra rich moisturizer (use a balm if your skin is extremely dehydrated) and a tinted moisturizer to even out skin tone. Do not use grainy scrubs or skin creams containing AHAs. Do not wear blush. Drink plenty of water as soon as you get up in the morning. Using a liter bottle to drink from rather than a glass seems to encourage me to drink larger quantities. (Consult with your doctor if your sunburn is severe. Aspirin may help with the inflammation.)

Quick Beauty Solutions

- Go to a hair salon and have your hair washed and blow-dried. (Even if you don't have an appointment, most salons will work you into their schedule.) Getting your hair to look good will make you feel more in control.
- Get a manicure. When I'm having a bad day, my husband sometimes suggests just this. He knows it always makes me feel better. If you are short on time or do not like wearing nail polish, consider having your nails buffed.
- Stop by a massage center and get a ten-minute neck and shoulder massage.

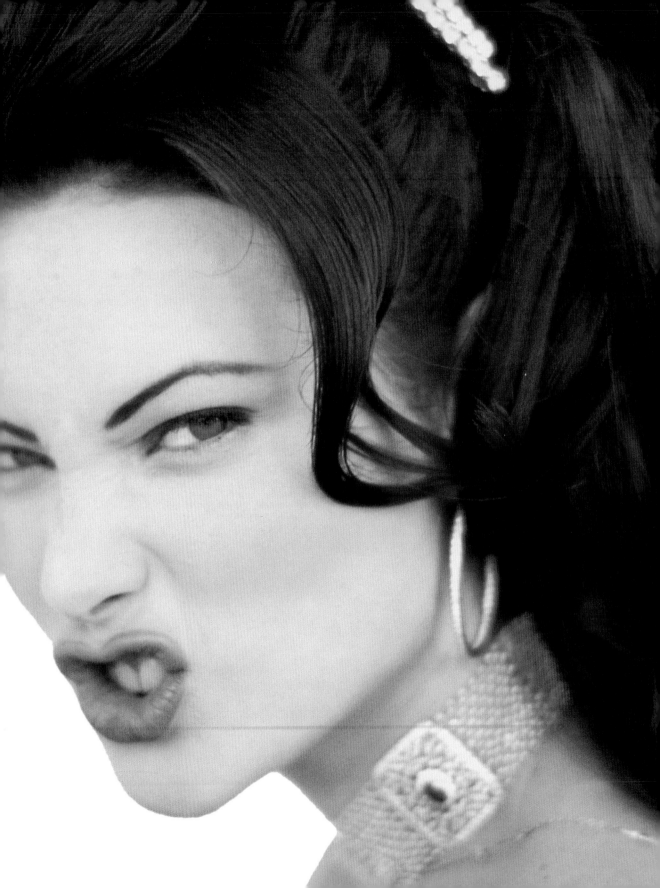

30

BAD-GIRL BEAUTY:
EXPERIMENTING WITH MAKEUP

Developing individual beauty style is the key to the makeup experience (see chapters 5, 6, and 7). But once you have defined that style, it is good occasionally to step out of the boundaries and do something out of character. It is fun to role-play and exciting to witness others looking at you differently.

These are the times to just have fun with makeup. I remind myself all the time: This isn't brain surgery; it is only makeup, and the minute it stops working, it can easily be washed off.

The reality is that most of us just want to get out the door looking good. But each of us should find moments to try new things without looking like a fashion victim. So go ahead and experiment with smoky eyes or red lip gloss. Wear it out or wipe it off. Red nail polish is flashy and fun and still noncommittal. Nail extensions, false eyelashes, a pale mouth, and liquid liner are all good ways to act out with your makeup. Look at magazines and get inspirations.

Where to draw the line? If you have to ask friends or family if you look silly, you probably do. Even at the age of three, my son tells me, "Mom, your makeup looks bad." I guess he's heard his father say just that!

It's highly individual. For me, just wearing eyeliner and mascara during the day is extreme. People react with surprise and tell me I'm wearing a lot of makeup. If I ever showed up in my office with red lips, it'd be talked about for months. There is nothing sexier or more modern than a clean face, charcoal liner, white highlighter, nude lip pencil, and white gloss.

And there need not be a special occasion to provoke you. It's as simple as wearing brown eyeliner to work if that's something you normally would never consider. After all, doing it when it's least expected is part of the fun!

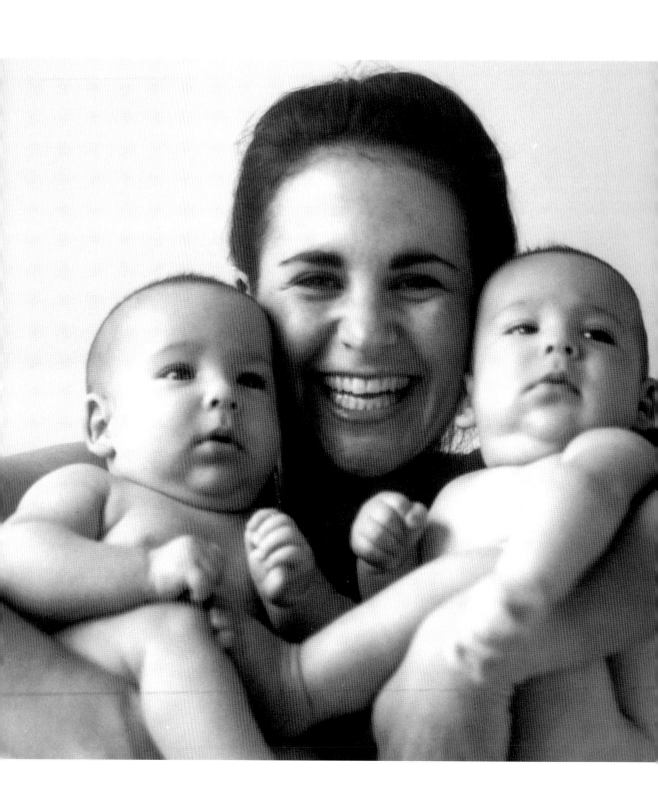

31

BEAUTY FOR PREGNANT WOMEN AND NEW MOTHERS

Being pregnant is an exciting, emotional time. Yet no matter how blissful you feel about becoming a mother, the fact is, you have lost control of your body. In the course of my two pregnancies, makeup became incredibly important to me as a means of feeling pretty and in control.

Exercising is another great way of maintaining a sense of control. I continued exercising throughout both of my pregnancies. Even if you just walk regularly, it will improve your mood and your body image. Pregnancy should not be an excuse to eat everything in sight and to stop moving. Continue to eat healthfully and drink lots of water.

There are no rules for pregnancy makeup. You can go pretty in pink makeup. Or, you can go sexy and dramatic—dark nails and lips are a great look on a pregnant woman. When you feel blue, be sure to wear blush. A light, clean scent can lift your mood, too.

The "Glow"

When you are visibly pregnant, people love to comment, "You've got that glow!" The truth is that during my two pregnancies, I didn't often have that glow naturally—it usually came from blush or bronzing powder. If you, like me, don't have that flushed, glowing look, there's no better time to get good with blush. (See chapter 14.)

Hair Coloring

Doctors usually recommend avoiding chemical hair dyes during the first three months of pregnancy—which is what I did. But I did go back to permanent coloring to cover my gray in the second trimester.

Many alternatives, however, do exist: Natural color rinses like henna (available in reddish and brown tones from health-food stores) are the safest choice; the pull-through method of streaking, which requires the wearing of a rubber cap over the scalp, is also considered very low-risk. Before doing any hair-coloring processes, advise your hair colorist that you are pregnant and consult your obstetrician.

Body Care

This is an important time to pamper yourself. Your body is going through extreme hormonal and physical changes, so you definitely deserve some special attention. What's more, once there's a baby in the picture, you will have little time for even the most basic beauty maintenance.

Treat yourself to massages. Look for a massage therapist who specializes in pregnancy. If you have a hard time spending the money on yourself, rationalize it this way: Instead of buying a shirt or a pair of shoes, you are getting a massage.

If you plan on wearing a swimsuit, don't forget to deal with your bikini line—it's still there even if you can't see it. Get a bikini wax.

Take care of your hands and feet—two parts of your body that don't change radically in pregnancy. If you are pregnant during the summer, paint your toenails and wear sandals.

Skin often becomes extremely dry during pregnancy. To soften and hydrate, put oil in the bath or rub oil onto your skin during showers. I especially like apricot oil in bathwater, but given that one's sense of smell is acute in these months, be sure to select a fragrance you find pleasing (or purchase nonscented bath oil).

Out of the bath, it's also nice to rub oil onto the body—especially over the breasts and abdomen. I had an amazing massage during my first pregnancy during which the therapist used a combination of cocoa butter and balm. It not only feels good, but it might help minimize the appearance of stretch marks. Of course, stretch marks are to a large extent hereditary and beyond our control. Nonetheless, why not do everything in our power to avoid them?

While some women claim their skin is at its most beautiful during pregnancy, others experience hormonal breakouts during pregnancy. Talk to your dermatologist if you can't manage your skin.

Note: "Mask of pregnancy" is a brown pigment that some women experience on their faces during pregnancy. It is caused by hormonal changes and is completely normal and will probably go away after you give birth. Consult your doctor if you are concerned.

Maternity Style

When I was pregnant, I made it a point not to wear maternity clothes. Why? Well, they are quite expensive and are useful only for a short time. And the cutesy look of most maternity clothes (i.e., Peter Pan collars, overfeminine prints, and bows) is off-putting to me.

Instead, I raided my husband's wardrobe for his crisp white shirts. I also purchased a men's jacket at a secondhand clothing shop and large-size button-down Oxford shirts at the Gap. I did, however, purchase leggings and jeans with "pregnancy panels" at a maternity clothing shop. One of my favorite looks from my third trimester was a black unitard (which creates a great long line) with a blazer worn on top. I wore my hair in a ponytail with "grown-up" polished makeup.

Many pregnant women chop off all their hair out of frustration with their looks. Try to resist making a drastic or impulsive hair change—you might feel miserably unfeminine about it later on.

Packing for the Hospital

Create a mini beauty kit containing sheer or natural lipstick, a blush, and concealer. You will be happy to be able to touch up when visitors start stopping by and flashes start popping. Even un-made-up and tired, you will cherish hospital pictures of you and your newborn. Also, take along a favorite moisturizer and cleanser. Leave perfume and scented lotions at home.

Home with Baby

First Few Days: When you first arrive at home with the baby, you won't be able to think about your looks. This is not a time to be lining your lips or curling your lashes. Accept that this period will be a blur and go with it.

First Week: Once you have established something of a routine, try to work in a minimal makeup look. Choose three things, such as concealer, blush, and lipstick; eyebrows, blush, and lipstick; or mascara, concealer, and lipstick, and take the extra time to do these steps. Be happy that you have managed to get dressed and get your look pulled together. (See chapter 19.)

It is easy to get caught in the trap of not dressing and not bathing—suddenly you realize it's 2:30 in the afternoon and you are still wearing your PJs. Try to force yourself to shower and dress when it's clear that you are up for the day. A shower (if you can manage) will make you feel fresh. If you can't manage to squeeze in your beauty routine when you first get up, you may never again find the opportunity.

Weeks That Follow: It's time to start spending a little more time on yourself. Go for a haircut or trim or a wash and blow-dry. Get a manicure or a massage. After about six weeks, return to your fitness routine. There will be lots of demands on your time and energy—the baby needs you and your husband needs you—but no one will benefit if you neglect yourself.

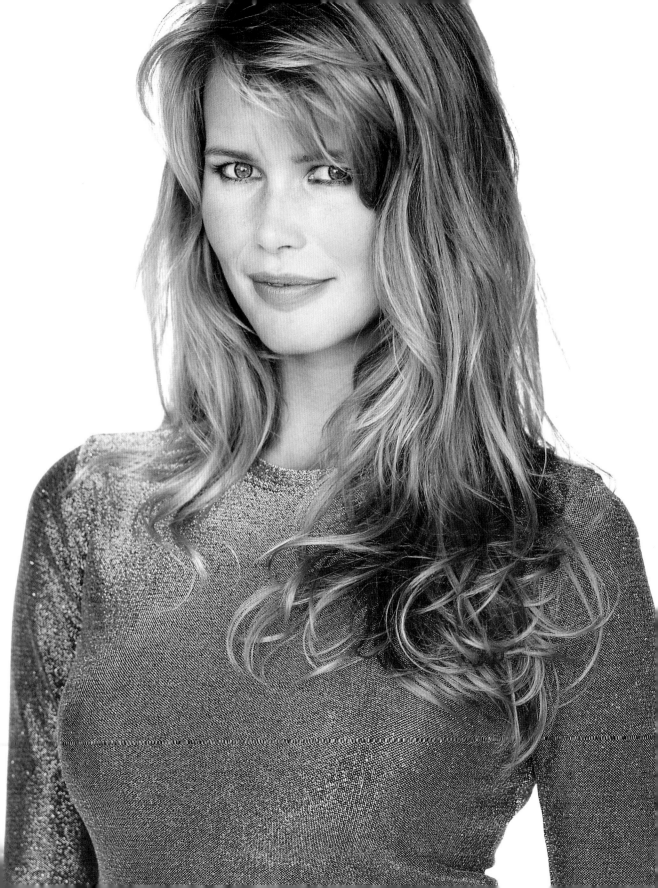

32

BLACK-TIE BEAUTY

Simplicity is the key to dressed-up beauty style: Heavy makeup just doesn't look modern or sophisticated. What's more, if you typically don't wear a lot of makeup, you will not feel like yourself when you do serious make-up. Going from A to Z for a special event is never a good idea. Most of us have memories of a glaring prom disaster to remind us of this.

Foundation should be the same for day and night. Some women try to create a porcelain finish on face and neck for evening by using a paler foundation than usual. I think that's a mistake: It's always correct and modern to match your skin tone.

Shadow, Mascara, and Color

The basic idea for evening is to wear cooler colors like white, gray, charcoal, and black instead of warmer, "day" tones like vanilla, taupe, and bone. Cooler colors are more dressy because they are in stronger contrast to your skin tone.

	Day	Evening
shadow	brown	gray
liner	brown	charcoal
highlighter	bone	white
mascara	brown	black (2–3 layers)
eye look	clean	smoky

Lips

This is the obvious place to go for glamour, if that's what you want. Reds and burgundies always look right for night. It is also modern and equally elegant not to do a big colorful lip, i.e., to match the natural color of your lip, as you would do for day, then go for a slightly richer or more deeply pigmented color for night. Or you can play with the finish: Go slightly more shimmery, darker, or lighter. Layering matte lip color with shimmer or gloss is beautiful for night.

If, however, you like to wear bright lipsticks by day, go ahead and wear bright lip colors at night. Experiment to heighten the effect. Go brighter yet or mix your bright lipstick with a darker pencil.

For a black-tie affair, you will want to pay much closer attention to the application of lip color.

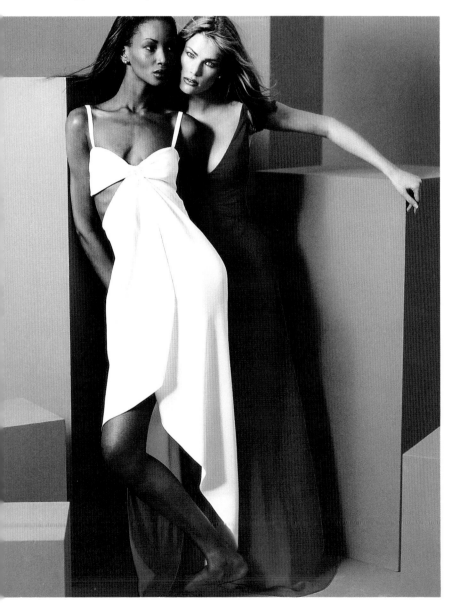

Tips

- Be sure to use a lip pencil; try going a shade darker than your usual day shade.

     Note: Lip pencil will help keep lip color in place and assure longer wear.

- Do a heavier application of lipstick than you would during the day.

- This is a good opportunity to use a lip brush, especially if color is intense.

Powder

Powder is essential for a polished, finished evening face. Powder around the eye to set concealer, and powder your face to set foundation, creamy blush, and pencils.

Note: Some makeup artists suggest holding a tissue up to your mouth and dusting powder over it, so that a little powder filters through to set lip color. I don't recommend this technique since it can thicken and clot the creamy texture of your lipstick.

Black-Tie Tips

- If your neck and chest are exposed, use a wide brush to apply a light bronzing powder or dark face powder. Blend downward from chin to avoid an obvious line. Note: Don't apply foundation on your neck or chest; you risk creating streaks or staining clothes.

- If your arms and chest are exposed in the middle of winter, check that your foundation doesn't make your face visibly darker than your exposed skin. It's a good idea to have a lighter foundation shade on hand in your paler months.

- Moisturize all exposed parts: arms, chest, neck, and, in summer, legs—especially calves and heels—with a rich cream for a healthy, creamy look to skin.

- I think the most elegant nail look for night is short: Red or dark colors are always right, as are the newer pale shimmers and opalescent enamels.

Black-Tie Mistakes

- Gold or silver shimmer powder that is dusted over shoulder or chest is a definite mistake—it looks cheap.

- Overelaborate hairstyles tend to look old-fashioned. Keep your hair shiny and touchable.

- Anything overrevealing or constraining; resist all attempts to look like a Cosmo cover girl.

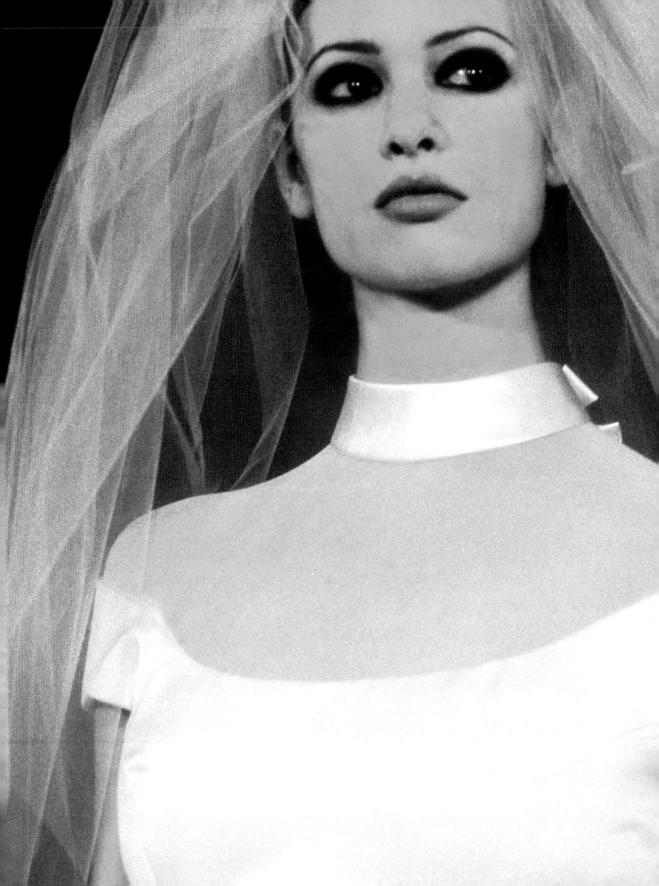

33

BRIDAL BEAUTY

The big day is in on the calendar. You're in search of the perfect dress, the perfect invitation, the perfect photographer, the perfect party place, the perfect flowers, the perfect music. You've got to think about calligraphers, napkins, cakes, and his difficult aunt Cecilia. Oh, yes, there's just one more thing: your face.

Wedding-day beauty should be a priority. This is the one day of your life when you are guaranteed to be the star attraction. It's natural to feel pressure to look beautiful since it's a given that everyone will be scrutinizing you. What is the most beautiful, appropriate bridal beauty? It's you at your most gorgeous.

WEDDING MAKEUP

This is not the moment to try anything tricky or novel, nor is it a time to experiment with the makeup look of the moment. Makeup trends change as quickly as fashion ones—the last thing you want is to be trapped in this moment's trendy makeup in the photographs in your wedding album. Chances are you'll regret it.

Do your makeup as if you were going to a black-tie event. Everything should be stronger and pretty, even if it is a day wedding. (Refer to long-lasting makeup techniques, chapter 18, and makeup for photography, chapter 24.)

- Wear a pretty shade of blush—pink if you are fair, rose if you are dark. Use slightly more than you usually do.
- Apply waterproof mascara, as it will last longer and withstand tears.
- Use white shadow as highlighter on your brow bone if you have light skin; a warm, light peach or vanilla highlighter if you have dark skin. This is a great look with wedding dresses.
- Charcoal, navy, or mahogany are nice options for eyeliner. In general, keep shadow colors light to medium.
- This would be a nice occasion to contour your eyes slightly, but avoid

using a strong color like charcoal so that your eyes do not appear to be too recessed (for contouring technique, see chapter 13).

- Be sure to define brows, but don't make them overpowering.
- Pale or brown lip colors can wash out your face in pictures, particularly when you are wearing white. It is a good idea to brighten lip shade slightly. If you normally wear brown or neutral, wear that as your base and put a pink or rose color on top. Or use your normal neutral lipstick with a brighter lip pencil, such as pink. On the other hand, if you normally wear dark lipstick, use that as your base and apply a lighter pink on top to give you a lift.
- You may mix various lip colors when applying makeup, but be sure to have one great lipstick color to carry with you for touch-ups.
- Use bronzing powder on your neck and chest if you need to even out your skin color. You don't want your face to appear to be a different shade than the rest of you. Do not use foundation on your chest: It can stain your dress.
- Avoid frosted makeup, since it creases easily and is too reflective for photographs.

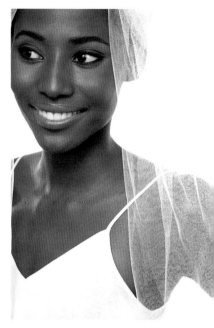

Wedding-Day Carry-Alongs

Give the following items to a bridesmaid or your maid of honor.

Loose Powder and Velour Powder Puff: You don't want your face to look shiny in the pictures. Make sure you ask your mother or bridesmaid to keep an eye on your shine quotient. Even a little shine will look like a greasy glow in pictures.

Lipstick: Keep it simple—choose one flattering color that you love.

Tissues and/or Cotton or Lace Handkerchief

De-Reddening Eyedrops: Even if you don't expect to cry.

Fragrance: A purse size of the scent you are wearing.

Wedding-Day Scent

Choose a fragrance that you really love and layer it so that it will stay with you all through the day. By layering different concentrations and formulations of your scent, it will never be overpowering.

After you shower, apply your fragrance's body lotion on your still damp skin—all over your body. Next, dot its perfume on your pulse points—behind knees, at wrists, on ankle bones, and behind the ears.

HIRING A MAKEUP ARTIST

You would like to hire a makeup artist to do your wedding face, but how do you find someone qualified? Ask friends who have had their makeup done for a big event. Inquire at the makeup counters at local department stores or beauty salons. Sometimes the salespeople behind the counters are also quite capable makeup artists. You might also phone a local modeling school for suggestions.

Before deciding on the makeup artist, speak to him/her: Ask if he/she has ever done makeup for a wedding. Ask to see pictures of his/her work. Request that you do a complete dry run of the wedding makeup a week or two before the event so that you are sure you like the look. If you meet with any resistance on doing a dry run, move on to the next name on your list. Hiring a makeup artist without trying him or her first could lead to a disaster! Discuss fees and dates up-front so that there are no misunderstandings. Remember to allow one solid hour for both the dry run and the actual wedding-day application.

If you cannot afford or cannot find someone in your area, arrange to go to a department store to have a makeup lesson. Then practice the look. Do your own run-through a week or so before the wedding. Arrange to have your maid of honor or a bridesmaid there with you to help critique your job.

HAIR

Lots of women choose to do complex, extravagant hairstyles for their weddings. If that's what you like, this is definitely the moment to go for it. As with your makeup, be sure to do a dry run with your hairstylists in the weeks before the wedding to work out the exact style you want. Be sure to bring your headpiece or veil with you to the salon.

Yet before you commit to a fantasy hairdo, consider a more simple and classic approach. Hair that's worn down is gorgeous. A simple, sleek ponytail can also be lovely. It is important to feel like yourself, not like an actress dressed up for a part in a period movie or the image your mother has for you on your wedding day.

SKIN

Planning a wedding is fun and exciting, but it is inevitably stressful, too. And stress can wreck havoc with your skin. Start taking extra good care of yourself as soon as possible. Get the sleep you need, proper nutrition, and drink plenty of water. Exercise regularly. Go for long walks. Do anything you can to keep stress at bay.

This is a good time to become a master of concealer (see chapter 11) and to learn to layer foundation on blemishes and to set with powder. **Wedding Week De-Stressing Techniques:** Get a massage. Take a bath. Go for a run the morning of your wedding. Do whatever works for you to calm yourself. Try not to be so swept up in the occasion that you lose sight of what's really going on.

NAILS

Sheer pink is a pretty choice for your nails. It looks fresh and is easy to touch up. Even if it chips, it won't be noticeable. Treat yourself to a manicure (and a pedicure, especially if you are going on a beach honeymoon).

TROUBLESHOOTING: HOW NOT TO SABOTAGE YOUR WEDDING LOOKS

- Unless you routinely get facials and never have a bad reaction, don't get a facial in the week before the event.
- Avoid getting too much sun just before the wedding. A red face is never attractive in a picture. And tan lines might look silly with your dress.
- Do not get a big-change haircut or new hair color in the weeks leading up to your marriage.
- If you have a blemish or a breakout just before your day, keep your hands off your face. Don't pick, squeeze, or attack. Your face will look just fine if you just leave things alone. (In the case of an emergency glaring pimple, see your dermatologiot.)

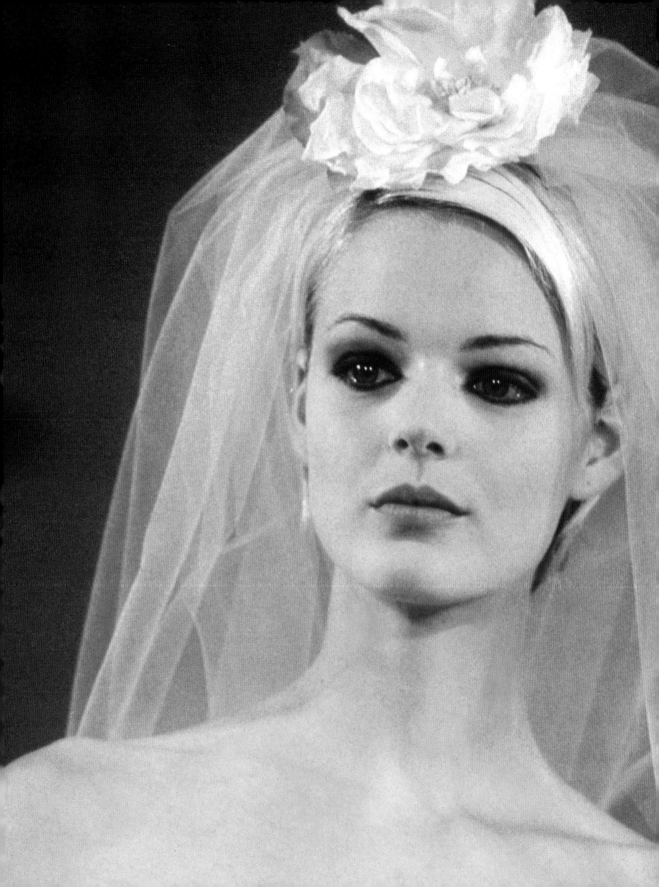

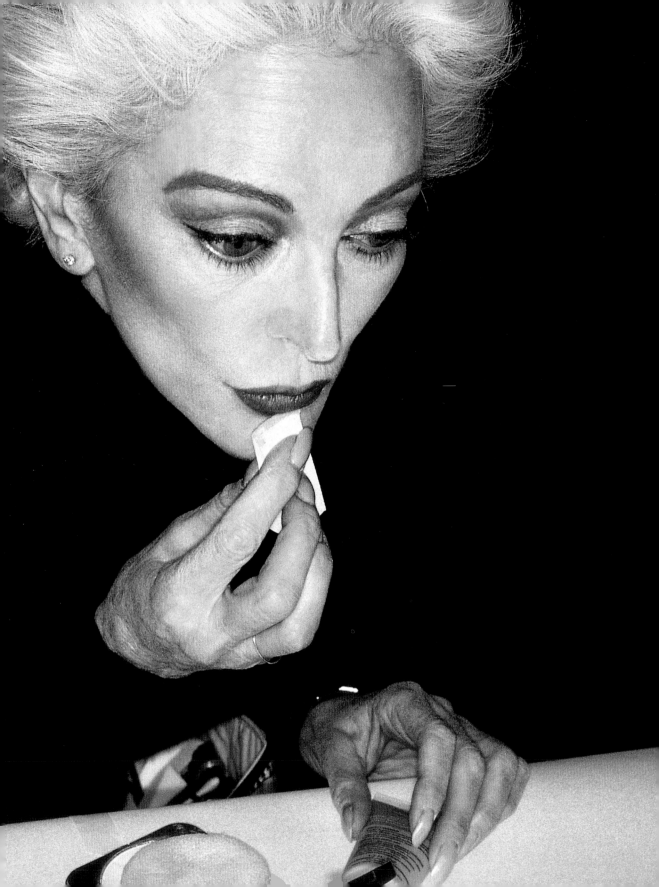

34

40+/50+ BEAUTY

40+: Prime Years

Turning forty is often traumatic. Many associate the number with loss of youth or the beginning of middle age. Nothing could be further from the truth. Age forty today is much younger than it was for your mother or grandmother. The forties decade now represents a time when women can be their strongest, most vibrant, independent, and sexy. (Think of all the Hollywood leading ladies and female rock stars in their forties!)

While in our thirties, many of us are focused on careers and family and how to juggle those two elements of our lives. Conversely, in our forties there is finally some time for ourselves. The kids are probably school age or older. One's career is probably in its groove. If you have been a stay-at-home mom, maybe it's the moment you choose to go back to work. You have developed a strong sense of self. You have accepted your body and now there's probably more opportunity than ever to exercise and get into the best possible shape. Perhaps there's more money for a nicer wardrobe or a trip to a spa. Whatever you do, be positive about this time; you'll look and feel your best.

50+ Beauty Style

Good health and natural beauty have always gone hand in hand. The link between one's health and looks becomes more apparent with the passing of years. Over-fifty beauty is based on taking care of yourself: eating healthy foods, drinking lots of water, wearing sunblock, and taking care to go to the doctor for regular physicals, yearly mammograms, etc. More than ever, beauty at this time of your life is based on feeling good about yourself.

It is a fact of life that as you get older, you lose color in your lips and your face. Gravity takes it toll on your face and your body. Exercise is one sure way to bring color into your face and make you feel and look your youngest. It is never too late to start a fitness program—join a gym, take a class at the Y, or inquire whether there is mall-walking club at your local shopping center.

This is also a time to simplify your style—both in clothes and makeup. I often find that with women in their fifties, sixties, and seventies it is their energy, smiles, and happiness that are their miracle cosmetics. Be sure to wear comfortable shoes—there's nothing more youthful than walking around in boat shoes or Keds. Find a simple, low-maintenance hairstyle. Develop a style that is right for your age—not the braids and overalls that would suit your granddaughter, and not the bun and shapeless clothes that remind you of your grandmother.

Sun: If you live in a warm climate (or spend time in one), be careful not to get too much sun. A leathery appearance to the face is aging and never attractive. If you like a tanned look, learn to use bronzing powder instead. (See chapter 14.) Whenever you are outside, be sure to wear sunblock on chest and hands, too.

Blending: Be extra careful to blend foundation up into your hairline and down over your jawbone. Find the sunniest spot in your home to double-check your makeup; using a hand mirror, make sure your makeup is well blended. Wear your glasses when applying makeup. Make a point of checking that your foundation is a perfect match to your skin tone every six months or so. The most careful blending in the world will not fix the wrong color foundation.

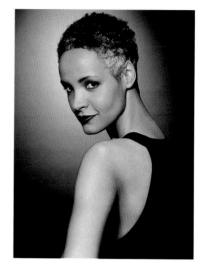

Makeup for Dry Skin: Use a moisturizer that isn't too greasy but that hydrates skin well. Wear moisturizing foundation (with yellow undertones) and make sure that your face powder is silky and light. Wear cream eye shadows, creamy lipsticks, and cream blushes. The trick is to apply cream blush just after foundation. Then dust on face powder. Apply a pop of powder blush on top.

Lipstick Feathering: To avoid feathering, line your mouth with a lip pencil, or apply powder over foundation and just above lip line to prevent color from running.

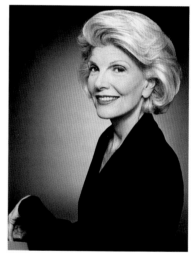

Lines: The older women I most admire are those who wear their wrinkles well—Helen Hayes was my all-time favorite beauty. These are women who are satisfied with themselves from the inside of their souls. They don't know the name of the best plastic surgeon in town, and they don't obsess over every little line they discover when looking in the mirror. They garden and walk and have a strong purpose to their lives. And they are beautiful and happy!

Your grandmother may have instinctually known that religious avoidance of the sun and cigarettes were the best ways to avoid wrinkles. Science has proven her right.

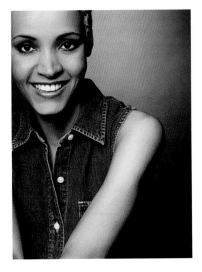

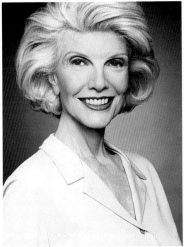

Plastic Surgery: I recommend considering this option only when, in the pit of your stomach, you are completely distressed over a feature. So often I recognize that a woman has had a face-lift, and I ask myself: What is the point of having a tight face when your neck and hands stay the same? It doesn't look right to my eye.

Question: Is there a good way to minimize the look of my crow's-feet?

Answer: Moisturizing your face regularly and drinking plenty of water will help give a smoother, plumper appearance to your face. Eye cream, which is normally slightly richer than face cream, is probably a good idea all around your eye area, both in the morning and at night.

The cause of crow's-feet is twofold: First, there is a genetic component; second, they are a result of years of smiling. So, the way I look at it, how can they possibly be bad?

Note: A brighter blush will take attention away from the eye area.

Question: Do women need more or less makeup as they get older, say, from age forty to sixty?

Answer: It is perhaps more a question of the *kind of* makeup rather than its quantity. Our natural coloring fades as we age: Lip color becomes less pronounced, skin tone becomes less vibrant. It is important to wear a bit more subtle color, such as more vibrant blush and lipstick colors, to avoid looking washed-out. (Brown lipstick is a bad idea for an older woman.) Also, since skin becomes drier with age, richer moisturizers and foundations are warranted.

Question: What are the best makeup tricks for playing down wrinkles?

Answer: The best makeup advice is to play up your strongest feature. Beyond that, it is important to keep skin extremely well moisturized and to wear a hydrating formula foundation.

Question: What can I do about the brown spots on my face?

Answer: Use sunblock daily to prevent any additional spots from forming. For existing brown spots, you may want to explore lightening creams. They do work, but they require a long time to see results.

Ask your dermatologist about techniques to remove spots.

Brown Spots

How to Prevent Them: Diligent use of sunblock is essential for prevention.

How to Conceal Them: Apply concealer (one tone lighter than skin tone) with a concealer brush to cover brown spots. Then apply foundation all over face. Be careful to use a gentle touch over the areas you have already concealed. Let foundation absorb for thirty seconds. Then, if necessary, apply more concealer on any remaining visible spots. Set with powder.

Concealing brown spots is easier if skin is well hydrated.

How to Fade/Remove Them: Over-the-counter skin lighteners do work to fade brown spots but require an extended treatment period before results are visible. The other option is to consult a dermatologist about having spots chemically lightened.

EYEGLASSES AND YOUR BEAUTY

For lots of women, eyeglasses are an everyday reality. For others, it is an option on days when our eyes are too tired for contacts. Whichever category you identify with, the last thing you want to do is to let your beauty fade behind your eyeglasses.

One makeup casualty with eyeglasses is that the frames tend to rub away foundation. When you go to the ladies' room, take off your glasses and do a quick blend of foundation. It is also extra important to define your brow when wearing eyeglasses. Take an extra moment to fill in your brow with a brown-toned shadow so that your own eyebrow, rather than the glasses frames, is defining your face.

If your glasses are a bold red or green, that's enough color around the eyes. Focus instead on great lipstick. If you are sensitive or allergic to eye makeup, don't wear it. Instead, have a couple of different frames that you like and let that be your eye statement.

If your prescription minimizes your eyes, think about lining your eyes to try to make them stand out. It's probably a good idea to curl your lashes.

If your prescription maximizes your eyes, make sure that your mascara doesn't clump. Instead of doing a heavy-duty single coat of thickening mascara, try doing two coats of thinner, lengthening formula.

If you feel as if you disappear behind glasses, you might experiment by wearing more assertive types of frames. A heavy tortoise or black style looks surprisingly good even with fine features. It's a good idea to select frames when you have plenty of time to play around. Never go shopping for frames directly from an eye doctor's appointment if you have had dilating eyedrops; you cannot properly see yourself.

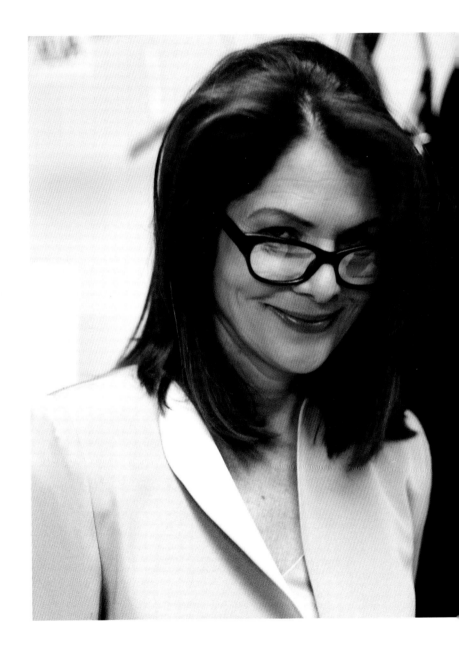

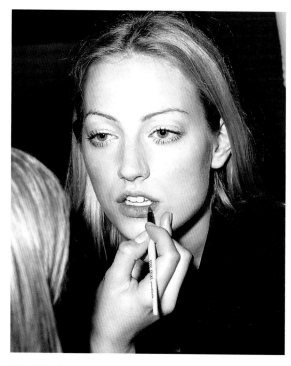
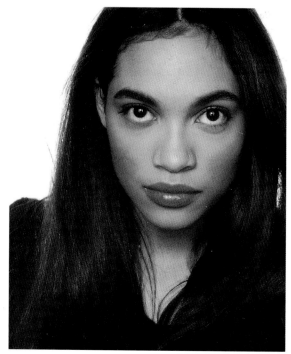
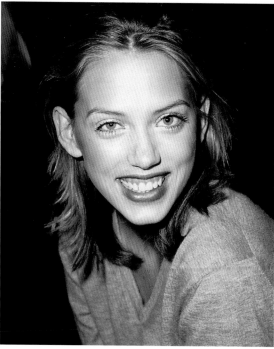
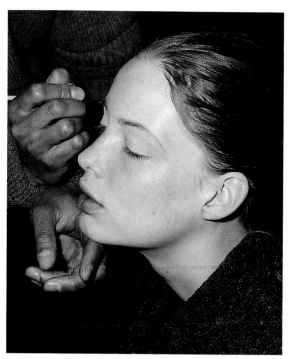

35

TEENAGE BEAUTY

This is the time to experiment with makeup—both in buying and in applying it. The two big issues are how much money should you spend, and how much makeup should you wear?

ETIQUETTE

I wouldn't recommend wearing makeup to school before high school. Lip gloss or tinted lip balm is fine for junior high school. Have fun finding fun colors and practicing with makeup at home with your friends. Going out in public heavily made up as a teenager is neither pretty nor appropriate. The best teenage beauty is pretty, fresh, and clean, never harsh. You don't want to look hard or as though you are trying to look older than you are. Red lips and black eyeliner will just end up looking silly.

MAKEUP BUDGET

The good news is that you don't need to spend a lot of money. The most inexpensive lipsticks, eye shadows, and nail polishes often come in the most creative colors. Makeup artists routinely find their most inspiring products at drug and dime stores—sometimes the very items that help them create a collection's look for the fashion runways. Maybe you'll want to treat yourself to one or two things at a department store, but there is no real need to spend the extra money.

PUTTING IT ON

The prettiest makeup look is based on light and sheer colors, like a pretty gloss and light, soft eye shadow shades. If you want to play with trendy colors, be sure to buy sheer versions of them so that they go on easily. You can also mix shadows with face powder to dilute them. Check out the makeup trends in fashion magazines like *Seventeen, Sassy*, and *YM* and experiment on your own face.

Avoid extremely dark or heavy makeup, such as black-lined lips or eyes and black nail polish—except on Halloween.

Concealer: Buy it to match your skin tone exactly. Use it to cover spots or blemishes. Blend it well so that it becomes invisible. I do not recommend using foundation.

Blush: Use cream or powder blushes in light shades.

Eye Shadows: Shimmery shadows can be pretty. Stick to pale shades or experiment with color. Avoid black.

Mascara: Brown is a good choice. You may want to experiment with other colors, though in the end you will probably come back to brown.

Lips: Use lip-colored lipsticks, lip gloss, sheer formulas, and stains.

SKIN CARE: CLEANSER PLUS MOISTURIZER

Your early teen years is the moment to establish your own skin-care ritual. It's time to find a cleanser that works for you. I recommend using a gel cleanser if you have oily skin or occasional breakouts. Bath soaps or detergent bar soaps are too harsh and drying for your face. Glycerin soaps are fine, especially if formulated for oily or sensitive skin. If your skin is dry, use a creamy cleanser. Cleanse your face both in the morning and at night, paying extra attention at the end of the day, when your face is grimier.

Moisturizing your face is also essential. Use an oil-free moisturizer if you are prone to breakouts. The tendency among teens who struggle with pimples is to overdry the skin. Drying out zits isn't the solution—really dry surface skin can end up trapping impurities beneath the skin, making matters worse. It is better to help your pores breathe via proper moisturizing. Pat on moisturizer when your skin is still slightly damp from cleansing, both in the morning and at night.

If blemishes are constantly present, consider going to a dermatologist. There are so many remedies available to you from a skin doctor that there is no reason to suffer with pimples, blackheads, or whiteheads. If you do not know a dermatologist, ask your school nurse or a friend. And as you've been told before, keep your hands off—picking at your face almost never makes things better. (See chapter 29 to learn how to cover a glaring pimple.)

Question: What can I do about blackheads? I wash and tone my skin and use masks, but I cannot get rid of them. Even after a professional facial, my blackheads are back in three weeks. Help!

Answer: Examine how you wash your face. Are you doing it in good light? Are you washing carefully along your hairline? If blackheads appear around the edges of your face, use a headband to pull back your hair and concentrate on cleaning these areas well. If blackheads appear on your nose and chin, try keeping a gentle grainy scrub in the shower (look for soothing ingredients like honey) and work scrub into affected areas two or three times a week.

Moisturizer containing alpha hydroxy acids sometimes help combat blackheads. Once a week, you may try steaming your face prior to cleansing it—it is helpful in keeping pores clean.

PROM MAKEUP

This is the appropriate moment to go slightly stronger with your look.
Concealer: Apply where needed and blend with your fingers.
Powder: Use a yellow-toned face powder, applied with a velour cotton puff, to even out your skin tone. Dust away excess.
Blush: Pretty, fresh cheeks (well-blended).
Eyes: Try plum, smoky, or gray shadows.
Mascara: Go for black.
Lips: Use a natural color lip pencil to outline lips together with shimmer gloss. If you keep your eyes natural, you may try a slightly stronger lip color.

Teen Scents

There is no need to spend a lot of money on fragrances. Nor is it suitable to wear powerful, strong scents. Look for fresh, lemony scents or single-note florals at your favorite drugstore. Stay away from oriental or heavy musk fragrances.

Test a scent first on your wrist. Since fragrances change with time, smell it thirty minutes later to see if you still like it before purchasing it.

BRACES

I spent four years in braces, so I can understand your frustration. Just remember that you will not regret the time spent in wires. Lips tend to get dry, so be sure to carry lip balm or gloss with you. Don't wear bright or loud colors on lips since that will draw extra attention to your mouth.

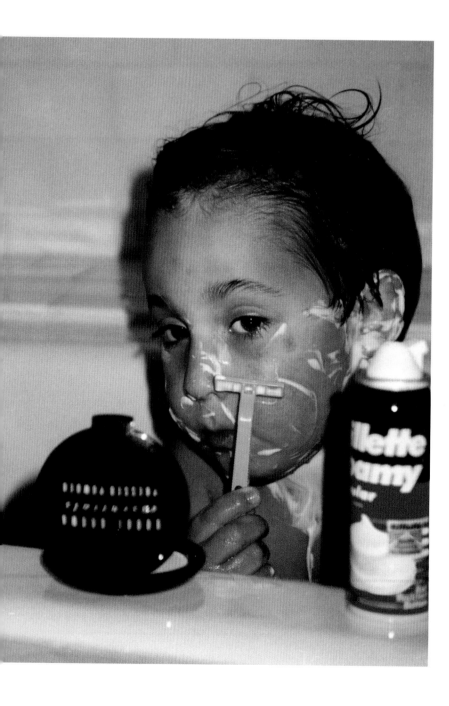

36

MEN AND GROOMING

Men's grooming is one of those taboo topics: Real guys don't use moisturizer. And the women in their lives accept this attitude while watching them borrow freely from their skin-care supplies (and the guys clearly enjoying it).

My message to guys: Why not look your best? All it takes is getting your grooming organized and figuring out the few products that you like and need. In the end, you will probably look younger and get out the door faster because of it.

Shaving: Wetting, steaming, and soaping the face with warm water are all necessary prep steps for a good shave. The best possible place to shave is in the shower, as it's an easy place to accomplish all that's necessary. (Finding a fog-free mirror that really works isn't always so easy.) I think shaving creams that come in a can are the best, but other options include the classic brush and shaving bar or shaving cream from a tube or jar.

Aftershave or toner will help close pores after shaving. (Cold water works, too.)

Skin Care: Having a good skin-care routine doesn't require lots of bottles and complicated steps. Cleansing and moisturizing are the two basic elements. Most men use bar soap on their bodies and faces. If that works for you, fine. But if you have sensitive skin or extremely dry or oily skin, you may want to find a more gentle cleansing cream or gel.

Find a good basic moisturizer (men usually prefer unscented formulas) for face and body. Apply when your skin is still damp from the shower.

Creams and lotions containing alpha hydroxy acids help smooth skin, and can even prevent blackheads and in-grown hairs.

Beware: Do not apply AHA skin lotions on just-shaved skin—it can burn.

Wear a heavier cream or balm on face for skiing or water sports.

It's hard to convince many sports-minded men of this, but a bright red face or neck doesn't look good on anyone. Wear a high-SPF sunblock whenever you are exposed to the sun and apply hydrating cream to your face and hands after sun exposure.

Nose Hair/Ear Hair: Use nose clippers or small electric nose shaver to nip protruding hairs. The same implement works to keep your sideburns and the hairline at your neck neat-looking between trips to the barber.

Eyebrows: If your eyebrows grow together above your nose (the mono-brow syndrome), consider waxing this small area. I don't think men should tweeze hairs above or below the brow line, as a man's own natural brow usually suits him best.

Body Waxing: The is a well-accepted option to remove hair on the back or chest. Go to a salon that does waxing for men.

Covering Gray: It's a great way to deduct years from your appearance. Use caution with at-home hair colorants, as they can be tricky to get right. It's probably best to go to a salon or barbershop in your city that does hair coloring for men. Start with a minimal amount of coverage to see if you like it.

A white mustache or beard can in some cases be charming and in others quite aging—if it's the latter, consider covering the gray or returning to a clean-faced look.

Men and Makeup

Rock stars wear makeup. I have done basic face powder on everyone from Bruce Springsteen and Bono to Sting and black eyeliner for Keith Richards. News anchormen, politicians, television personalities, stage actors, and male models all do some degree of making up. For those men whose work takes them onstage or in front of the camera, serious makeup is part of the job.

Does the average guy need to wear makeup to go to work? No—because looking rugged and natural is our society's definition of male good looks.

There are, however, more minimal measures that men can take when and if they choose and still look totally natural.

Self-Tanning Cream, Spray, or Gel: Activates your skin's own melanin to create a tanned look that lasts up to three or four days. Read all package directions and application tips in chapter 21 before undertaking.

Bronzing Powder or Gel: A cosmetic that gives warmer color to the face (be sure to wash palms after application). Some department-store lines have specific bronzing powders for men.

Concealer: For extremely black under-eye circles, use stick concealer that is one shade lighter than skin tone.

Foundation (Cream or Stick): Use to cover blemishes or red spots. It is important that foundation match your skin tone exactly.

Tinted Powder: For men with very oily skin, brush on powder that matches your skin tone to keep your face from becoming too shiny.

Brow Filler: Extremely pale or nonexistent eyebrows can be filled in with a small brush and a brown-toned shadow. Keep it light so it looks natural.

Lip Balm: Every guy can benefit from wearing lip balm, especially if outside doing sports.

Bobbi's Survey

How do guys feel about the makeup we wear? For the purposes of this book, we did a survey to find out. When asked their preference between pink and red lipstick, men chose red over pink by a three-to-one margin. Some qualified red as brown-toned reds while others seemed to prefer fire-engine reds. Others elaborated, saying that they felt pink tones were for older women.

The number-one biggest makeup turn-off? "Too much of it!" was the favorite answer. "Obvious and excessive makeup is the worst!" said one thirty-something man. "Overdoing it," said another. "Too much! Yuk!" exclaimed a twenty-eight-year-old guy. Cakey makeup was the next biggest turn-off: "Yucky, cakey makeup."

Men's Makeup Pet Peeves

- Too much of it
- Lipstick on her teeth
- Makeup that comes off on my face and my clothes
- Too-obvious blush that makes her look like a clown
- A visible line where makeup ends and skin begins
- Garish colors

The number-one biggest makeup turn-on? "Subtlety" was the most common response. "Makeup that makes a woman look more attractive," explained one. "Just the right amount—elegant yet real," said another. The men were evenly divided between preferring a more defined eye and a more defined lip. The majority noted specific makeup effects that they find pleasing, expressing themselves in rather personal, nontechnical terms.

Makeup Effects Men Find Attractive

- Moist lips
- Long lashes
- Wide-open eyes
- Dewy skin
- Sensual lip color

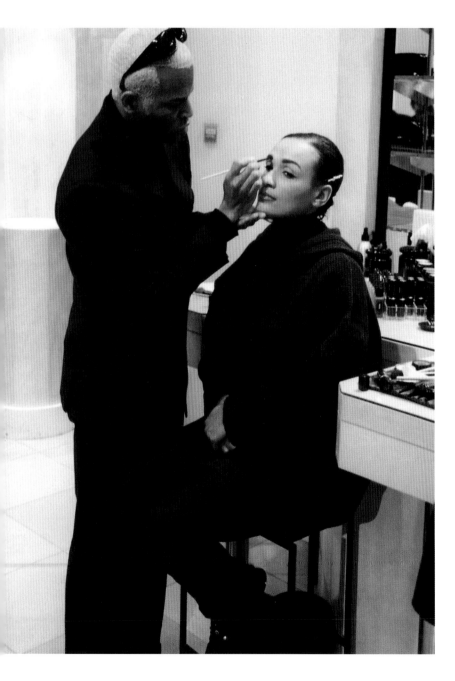

37

COUNTER INTELLIGENCE: SHOPPING FOR AND BUYING SKIN-CARE PRODUCTS AND MAKEUP

You Are Not a Victim

You step into a department store. A salesperson gloms on to you. You feel pressured. Your confidence starts slipping away. Makeup is suddenly being applied to your face. It is unlikely that—whatever your mission in entering the store—your real needs will be met. My advice? At the first sign of loss of control, walk away. Don't feel helpless. Don't find yourself saying, "She *made me* buy it." Just move on. It's happened to me—I am sometimes made to feel horrible when I shop for cosmetics—and I am sure most women can identify with this situation.

What I object to most is an attempt by salespeople to feed off your insecurities. Don't let anyone tell you that you look bad or ugly or moan on about your skin. No one needs that. It's also true that certain salespeople are under pressure to sell and add extra products on to what you had intended to purchase. Just remember that it's up to you whether you choose to give in to that pressure.

Instead of putting yourself at the mercy of a sales associate, take control of the situation. Be a tough critic. Ask yourself, for example, if this is a lip pencil you will really use. Can you visualize yourself applying this teal eye shadow? Analyze products carefully. If you are thinking about buying a cream, look at it. Do you like how it feels? How it smells? Be realistic: Is this something you will want to do every day? Is this a cream that will be fun to use? Or is this a product bound for the drawer at the bottom of your bathroom cabinet?

If you have to ask a friend's opinion of a lipstick, do not buy it. You should love it so much that you are compelled to purchase it!

Consumer Affairs

A lot of companies have samples of skin care, even lipsticks, and fragrance: Before committing to an expensive purchase, ask for a sample size and take it home.

Make a point to inspect the counter salespeople before approaching a counter. Approach a man or woman whose look you like—a person who seems friendly, kind, and helpful.

If you have a reaction to a product (especially a cream containing AHAs) or if the packaging is damaged in any way, take the product back to the counter where you bought it. Don't be embarrassed—most large cosmetic companies will accept returns if you are dissatisfied. If you meet with resistance, ask to speak to the manager of the store. Also, look on the back of the carton. Oftentimes there is an 800 number to call or addresses to write if you are not completely happy with the product.

Buying Tips/How Not to Waste Money on Makeup

- Keep cosmetics in a central area, so that you don't purchase things you already own. Edit your cache regularly.
- Women often buy lipstick (on impulse as a lift) only to arrive home to realize that they have the same basic shade from a variety of companies. If you indeed need a lipstick lift, make sure you break new ground with a darker, paler, or redder shade.
- Purchase the items you have the most difficulty with (i.e., finding foundation that really matches your skin tone) in an atmosphere where you can get the most help, like a department store or makeup shop.
- If you want a lot of attention, don't shop during high-traffic times, i.e., lunchtime (12–2 P.M.) or on Saturdays.
- Avoid gift-with-purchase colors or foundations. Chances are, they are not the perfect shades for you.
- Don't test foundation or concealer color on your hand. Match it to the skin on your face—where it will be worn. (See chapter 11.)
- Carry along a small mirror in your bag so that you can check how makeup looks. It is a good idea to step outside into natural light to judge whether a foundation matches.

The Makeup Marketplace

We would all love to live in the perfect one-stop-shop world. The truth is, we don't—not for our clothing wardrobes, not for our makeup wardrobes, and unfortunately, probably not even for tonight's family dinner. The most realistic approach is to surf among a variety of retail sectors, culling the best products and options from each.

Department-Store Makeup Counters: A great atmosphere to try new products, to match perfectly a foundation shade, to learn a new technique, or to smell the newest fragrance. What definitely to buy: foundation, concealer, and powder. What not necessarily to buy: trendy colors that you shouldn't spend a lot on.

Makeup Artists' Lines: Lots of professional makeup artists (including me) have launched their own lines, applying hands-on expertise to more advanced, and more modern product options than were previously available. Shop these lines for true yellow-toned foundations and powders, makeup brushes, beauty trends and news, compact-sized colors, and the most modern-looking packaging. Another plus are the young, usually well-trained makeup artists who work behind the counters.

Drugstores/Convenience Stores: The place to purchase beauty staples like cotton pads, latex sponges, Q-tips, and eyelash curlers inexpensively. Color cosmetic products to buy: lipsticks, lip pencils, eye pencils. What not to buy here: foundation, concealer, or powder—I feel you should be in an atmosphere where you can feel and touch these products so that you can find the perfect match with skin tone.

Health-Food Stores: A great place to find excellent creams (I often find much nicer creams at prices equivalent to those at drugstores). But because these products have fewer preservatives (that's part of the reason I like them), be especially careful to store them properly—away from heat and sunlight. Also check the packaging date and purchase from the most recent shipments. Some manufacturers recommend storing unopened creams, lotions, and sunblocks in the refrigerator.

Art-Supply Stores: The place to find the most beautiful (albeit expensive) brushes.

TV Infomercials: I do not recommend buying makeup or skin-care products that you can't see or try.

Catalogs, Store Flyers, Magazines: Beware of buying makeup colors from printed matter. It is extremely difficult to print cosmetic colors so that they are representative of the actual color. What you see is not always what you get. Mail order is convenient, however, when it comes to reordering products.

Quick and Free Beauty Boost

Feeling drab? Ask a counterperson to do an application of blush and lipstick. It only takes a minute but can give you a huge lift. The colors that the beauty associate chooses may reveal new options to you as well.

CONCLUSION

You could spend your entire life mastering all the makeup techniques I have detailed in this book. But please don't do that! I'd much prefer if you would use my makeup manual selectively, choosing the techniques and information most important to you. Then, at other moments or on another occasions, come back to the manual to pick up new information.

It's easier said than done, but try not to get caught up in the hype of the beauty world. Don't feel like you're the only one to have ever suffered through a bad beauty day—because, I promise you, we all have. Don't compare yourself to airbrushed images of perfection—because no one, anywhere, could ever look as good as the pictures we see in magazines.

When it comes to buying cosmetics, don't be cowed or pushed around by counter salespeople. Don't get frustrated if you don't get a new technique right on the first try—makeup, like anything else, takes a little practice. (Sometimes even for me!) And don't develop unrealistic expectations for products: There are no beauty miracles.

Strive to stay in control of your own beauty system. Develop your own individual beauty style: Look for the traits that make you special, learn to accentuate them, and then build your personal style around them. Learn to judge for yourself what works for you and what doesn't. Then, occasionally, just for the fun of it, break down and try something completely out of character. Remember: Makeup is not brain surgery—it washes away, so just have fun with it!

More than anything, I urge you to be positive and feel good about yourself. Perhaps it sounds clichéd to say that beauty starts on the inside, but this is one thing I have learned is an absolute truth. Feel confident, strong, and pretty on the inside. Then you will surely look pretty on the outside, too.

ADDENDUM I
MAKEUP ETIQUETTE

Perhaps it sounds old-fashioned to talk about makeup etiquette. Nonetheless, making up one's face is a social ritual and rules do exist. Whether you choose to consider or observe them is clearly up to you.

Applying lipstick and face powder is an accepted practice in public places—such as at a table in a restaurant. Personally, I prefer to wait until I am in a ladies' room since I feel self-conscious applying makeup in front of people. (Not surprisingly, I find that people like to analyze my technique, and sometimes I would just rather have a nice lunch and save the makeup lesson for later!) If you do choose to apply lipstick after dinner, do only a quick touch-up. If you have a reflective lipstick case, use that to check your application. Don't pull out a lip brush, compact mirror, and powder puff from your pocketbook for a painstaking process. Save that for the powder room (hence the name).

Using your morning commute to apply makeup might well allow you a few more minutes in bed, but it is definitely not a great idea. We should always be considerate of those around us, and public transportation is far too open a venue for your daily makeup routine. There are also risks involved in doing makeup on a moving vehicle. Should you come to a sudden stop, you could injure your eye with a mascara wand, tweezers, or a shadow brush. Instead, try getting up a few minutes earlier. You should be able to accomplish a finished look in five minutes or less.

Doing your makeup in the car is slightly more private and therefore more acceptable. We all are guilty of this from time to time. Whatever the circumstances, proper makeup etiquette centers on being discreet.

ADDENDUM II

MEDICAL CONSIDERATIONS: CHEMOTHERAPY MAKEUP AND CAMOUFLAGE TECHNIQUES

Makeup for Chemotherapy

Chemotherapy is a challenging, trying time for any woman. Besides the obvious emotional and medical issues you face, your physical appearance and identity is shifting and is seemingly out of your control.

I believe that this is a time not to abandon makeup altogether, as it can make you look and feel better about yourself. Nor is it a time to do serious or heavy makeup—it will look forced. Remember that this is a passing phase—your skin color will soon improve, and your hair will soon grow back. I recommend the following basic makeup routine:

- Use concealer, as needed, but be careful that the shade is not too light.
- Apply tinted moisturizer or foundation to give your skin a glow. Be sure that the shade is not too light or pasty.
- Fill in eyebrows—or create a brow line if you have lost the hair here—with a soft pencil. Go over brow line with shadow, using an eyeliner brush. If you have lost hair in spots, fill in just those areas.
- Use medium to soft browns on the eyes.
- If your eyelashes are sparse, use a slightly darker, smoky, powder liner along the lash line. This will create the illusion of lashes.
- Brush on a soft pink or rosy blush for a lift.
- Use flattering, warm lip shades, like rose, pink, or apricot.

Question: I am in chemotherapy and have lost my eyelashes. What can I do?
Answer: Your eyelashes are sure to begin growing back as soon as you complete your therapy. In the meantime, try this technique to give you the look of mascara: Using a liner brush and a smoky shade of shadow, line your eye as close to the lash line as possible. Do both top and bottom, using slightly more shadow on top lid. (See chapter 21.)

Look Good, Feel Better is a nationwide program that helps women undergoing chemotherapy deal with their looks. For information, call 404-329-5763.

Extreme Beauty Measures

Covering Scars: I love scars. I think they communicate a strong character. If, however, you choose to try to cover a facial scar, know from the onset that it is almost impossible to cover it 100 percent. You can make it much less obvious with makeup and also by playing up lips or eyes or cheeks.

Use your normal concealer or creamy foundation. Or for more serious, longer-lasting coverage, buy a heavy-duty concealer. Lydia O'Leary and CoverMark are two good lines that are sold at department stores.

Keloid (or Raised) Scar: The center of a scar is typically lighter or pinker than the rest of skin. Use concealer that matches your skin tone to darken center area. If coverage is not adequate, try a slightly darker shade of concealer. Seal with powder in shade matching skin tone.

Recessed Scar: Fill in the scar to make skin look smooth and even. Layer thin coats of concealer, then set with skin-tone-colored powder.

Covering Port-Wine Stains: This is a difficult process, but women who have port-wine stains are experts at this technique. Below, the basic thinking, which involves three layers of concealer coverage:

- Layer 1: Pale yellow concealer that is five shades lighter than skin tone.
- Layer 2: Light beige concealer that is two shades lighter than skin tone.
- Layer 3: Concealer that matches skin tone or is one shade darker. Set with powder in a shade that matches skin tone.

ADDENDUM III

HOW TO BECOME A MAKEUP ARTIST

So you want to be a makeup artist. I am often asked how to become what I am and the answer varies, depending on exactly what kind of makeup artist you want to be. Whatever your exact career objective, be fore-warned: It is an extremely competitive field and there are a lot of starving makeup artists around. You have to absolutely love it since, even though it may seem glamorous from the outside, it is not an easy life. For those who are determined, the rewards are many. Prepare yourself for the considerable time and effort it takes to get there.

The best advice for a newcomer to the field is always to be open-minded. Learn from whomever you can (older, established makeup artists, photographers, counter salespeople) in whatever situation that presents itself. I know that part of the reason I made it was that I was always nice to everyone I met in the business. I took note of people's names and made a point of going back to visit editors and photographers to show them new work. I remember saying to an editor once: "You might not hire me this time—but you will next time." It was early on for me to make such a pre-diction. But she agreed with me. We were both right! (I ended up fixing her up with her husband, so I joke with her now that I paid her back.)

Options

Department-Store Makeup Artist: A great way to gain experience, no matter what your ultimate goal. Try to get a job with one of the newer makeup artists' lines. If you find yourself selling makeup much more than applying it, you are not in the right place.

Bridal Makeup Artist: Contact the better bridal shops in your area to see whether they use or recommend makeup artists. Meet those people to discuss a possible apprenticeship. If you have wedding-makeup experi-ence, make an appointment with the owner of the shop and take your bridal portfolio in to show her/him.

Salon Makeup Artist: Check with the better beauty salons in your area to see if they use a makeup artist. Offer to assist that person. If you have some experience, arrange to meet the salon manager to discuss doing makeup for clients.

Theatrical Makeup Artist: There are many fine theatrical makeup programs, including my alma mater, Emerson College, in Boston.

Cinematic Makeup Artist: Since Hollywood is the center of the film world, it makes sense to try to base yourself there. Try to be an apprentice of a makeup artist whose work you admire.

Fashion Makeup Artist: I tend not to recommend makeup schools that specialize in fashion/advertising work, as I do not like the techniques most of them employ. The best way to learn fashion makeup is to apprentice yourself to an artist you admire. There is no better way to learn and make contacts. Think of this as your university; even if you must borrow money and work for free for many months, it will be worth it.

Practice

The best way to learn is to open your eyes and look at women. Ask yourself why they look good. Note the colors that they use.

Do makeup on your family and friends just for fun, at first. Then do makeup for them for special occasions. Once you feel comfortable, volunteer your services as an assistant to a working makeup artist in your town.

Portfolio—Getting Started

Take pictures of your makeup—even if they are Polaroids of the friends you've made up. Assemble the pictures in a book. Then go to a modeling agency in your town. Offer your makeup services for a test shooting. (A test refers to a photography session where no one gets paid, but everyone gets experience.) Make sure to ask up-front for a choice of pictures.

Do laser photocopies of photos for your book rather than having prints made—since that is very expensive. Slides are more difficult for people to view and do not always show makeup well enough.

Take your book to local advertising agencies, modeling agencies, bridal houses, local magazines. The fact is that bigger cities have more work. New York, Los Angeles, and Chicago all have big markets.

PHOTOGRAPHY CREDITS

viii: Ken Robinson. xi: Ilan Rubin. 2–3: Jeff Licata. 6: Troy Word. 10: Dennis Golonka. 14: (left) Kevin Mancuso, (right) George Holz. 16: Ilan Rubin. 19: Ilan Rubin. 21: Troy Word; hair by Creighton for Robert Kree salon. 24: Arthur Elgort. 26: Antoine Verglas. Courtesy *Self*. Copyright © 1992 by Condé Nast Publications Inc. 31: Walter Chin. 35: Tatjana Patitz by Patrick Demarchelier. Courtesy *Vogue*. Copyright © 1988 by Condé Nast Publications Inc. 38, 40–41: Photofest and Star File Photo Ltd. 42: Ken Robinson. 45: (left) Dennis Golonka, (center and right) Ken Robinson. 47: Ken Robinson. 48: Ken Robinson. 50: Bruce Weber. 52: Michel Arnaud. 53: Bruce Weber. 54: Brigitte Lacombe. 55: Troy Word; hair by Creighton for Robert Kree salon. 56: Troy Word. 57: (left) Dickie Plofker, (right) Brigitte Lacombe. 58–59: Brigitte Lacombe. 60: Antoine Verglas; hair by Harry King. 61: Gilles Bensimon. 62: Walter Chin. 63: Antoine Verglas. 64: Antoine Verglas. 65: Sheila Metzner. 66: Troy Word; hair by Creighton for Robert Kree salon. 74: Ilan Rubin. 77: Ilan Rubin. 78: Ilan Rubin; hand model Laura Gens. 81: Ilan Rubin. 83: Ilan Rubin. 84: Troy Word; model Kristeen Arnold/IMG; hair by Michael Johnson for Marek. 86: Ilan Rubin. 89: Ilan Rubin. 91: Ilan Rubin. 93: Ilan Rubin. 94: Troy Word; model Lene Hall/American Model Management. 96: Troy Word; model Kristeen Arnold /IMG. 98: Ken Robinson. 99: Dennis Golonka. 101: Dennis Golonka. 103: Troy Word; model Kristeen Arnold/IMG; hair by Michael Johnson for Marek. 104: Antoine Verglas. 107: Troy Word; model Kristeen Arnold/IMG. 108: Ken Robinson. 109: Ken Robinson. 110: Antoine Verglas. 113: Ken Robinson. 114: Ken Robinson. 117: Ken Robinson. 118: Walter Chin. 120: Troy Word; model Kristeen Arnold/IMG. 123: Dan Lecca. 124: Troy Word; model Kristeen Arnold/IMG. 127: Ken Robinson. 128: Ken Robinson. 131: Ernesto Urdaneta. 132: Walter Chin. 136: Dennis Golonka. 138: Dennis Golonka. 140–141: Dennis Golonka. 142–143: Dennis Golonka. 150: Patrick Demarchelier. Courtesy *Vogue*. Copyright © 1988 by Condé Nast Publications Inc. 155: Walter Chin. 156: Walter Chin. 158: Patrick Demarchelier. 160–161: Walter Chin. 164–165: Ken Robinson. 168: Ilan Rubin. 172: Walter Chin. 175: Dennis Golonka. 176: Dennis Golonka. 182: Patrick Demarchelier. Courtesy *Vogue*. Copyright © 1989 by Condé Nast Publications Inc. 184–185: Ken Robinson. 186: (left) Dennis Golonka, (center and right) Ken Robinson. 187: Antoine Verglas. 188: Walter Chin. 190–191: Ken Robinson. 192: Sante D'Orazio. 194: Walter Chin. 196: Jeff Licata. 200: Arthur Elgort. 202: Mechthild OpGenOorth. 206: Walter Chin. 208: Walter Chin. 210: Courtesy of Vera Wang. 212: Troy Word; model Lene Hall/American Model Management; veil courtesy of Vera Wang. 215: Courtesy of Vera Wang. 216: Ken Robinson. 218–219: Troy Word; models (top) Nicky Kunz and (bottom) Gloria Barnes/Ford Women. 221: Dennis Golonka. 222: (left top and bottom) Ken Robinson, (right top and bottom) Troy Word; (top right) model Rosario Dawson/Pauline's; hair by Michael Johnson for Marek.